Medical Investigation 301

A Book to Advance PERSPICACITY in Students of Medicine Science

By Dr. Richard Griffith
Medical Investigation 301

A definition of **PERSPICACITY**
...having a deep insight into a
subject, akin to shrewdness.

Written by

Dr. Richard Griffith

Guilford, Vermont

and

Published by

Dr. Russ Hill

Laguna Beach, CA

Note to the Reader

Medical Investigation 101 introduced students potentially interested in a career in medical science to aspects of clinical thinking and information gathering. In Medical Investigation 301, the same authors, Dr. Richard Griffith and Dr. Russ Hill take this process one step further. Griffith will do all the writing this time with Hill acting as the editor-in-chief. Dr. Hill, a Podiatrist who later turned to teaching science in a California middle school, conceived the original idea to create materials to encourage interest in the medical sciences. He talked his cousin, Griffith, into contributing to the effort. In this new book, available on Amazon, we seek to create a more advanced perspective on medical science that we hope will enhance the reader's ability to enter a formal study of medical science in a way that puts them ahead of the pack. We also believe this perspective can prove provocative for any reader regardless of their career objectives.

What do we mean by a new perspective? Early in the Democratic presidential campaigns in 2020 Andrew Yang appeared on television wearing a MATH label pin. He intended his pin not to advocate mathematics, but to stand for a campaign theme of "Make America Think Harder." The word "Perspicacity" in the title of this book has a very similar intent. Faculty try to impart a massive amount of information to students of medical science to make them capable. This process can have the effect of overwhelming their ability to integrate and digest foundational concepts. In that sense, this book shares Andrew Yang's mission.

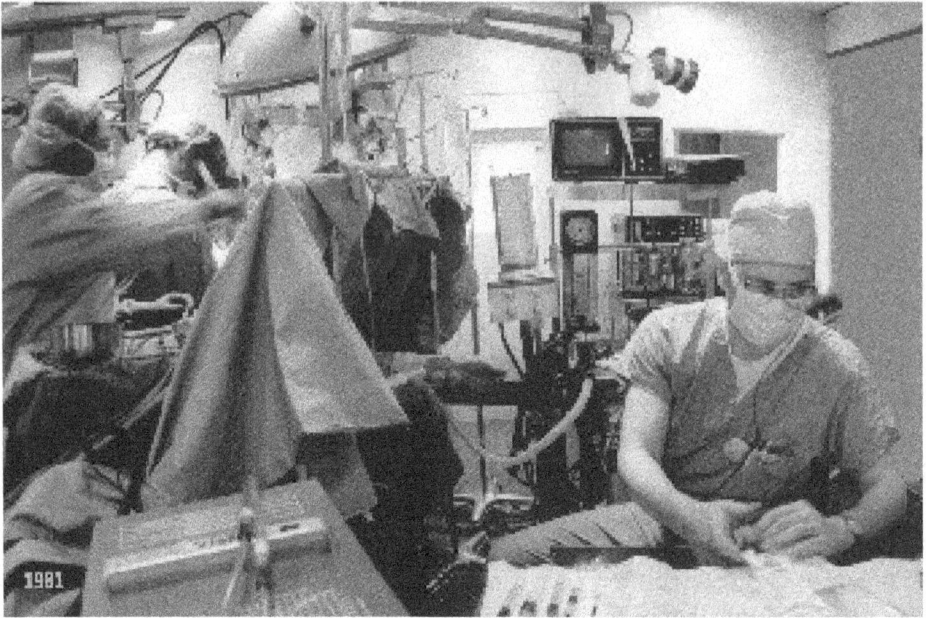

Dr. Griffith majored in physics in college and earned a Doctor of Science Degree in Electrical Engineering before attending medical school. Immediately after medical school he contributed his engineering skills for two years as a principal investigator in an NIH funded Head Trauma Center. He did a residency in anesthesiology and during his career practiced that specialty both in private practice and in an academic setting. He also spent a decade as a medical director in a Fortune 500 medical device company. He brings all of those experiences to this unusual take on the learning process for careers in healthcare.

You need not have read Medical Investigation 101 as a prerequisite for this book. We target in this volume an audience at a senior high school level and beyond. The number 301 signals that this material has a more complex content and a different focus than the earlier Medical Investigation 101 that introduced young students to medical science as a STEM subject.

Table of Contents

CHAPTER 1 THE FIREHOSE EFFECT.. 7

CHAPTER 2: BARRIERS TO MEDICAL EDUCATION..19

CHAPTER 3: THE CHEMISTRY OF LIFE 22

CHAPTER 4 THE MIRACLE OF COAGULATION...28

CHAPTER 5 WHY DO GERMS AND VIRUSES HATE US?.............................33

CHAPTER 6 CANCER 41

CHAPTER 7 CONTROL SYSTEMS 45

CHAPTER 8 TIME OUT 52

CHAPTER 9 HOW DOES THE BODY KNOW IT HAS BEEN INJURED?...............55

CHAPTER 10 MEDICAL MISADVENTURES 65

CHAPTER 11 PHYSICAL EXAMINATION 83

CHAPTER 12 WHAT IS A VIRUS?...88

CHAPTER 13 WHAT GOOD IS ANGINA? 93

CHAPTER 14 WHAT IS A FEVER?...98

CHAPTER 15 WHAT ARE WE GOING TO DO WITH GENETICS?....................102

CHAPTER 16 WHAT SHOULD WE EXPECT FROM ARTIFICIAL INTELLIGENCE?
....106

CHAPTER 17 THE CULMINATION...112

Chapter 1 The Firehose Effect

A three-inch firehose can efficiently deliver,
A 500 gallon per minute swift-running river.
That's much more than a drinking fountain spirts,
And to sip from a firehose just plain hurts.

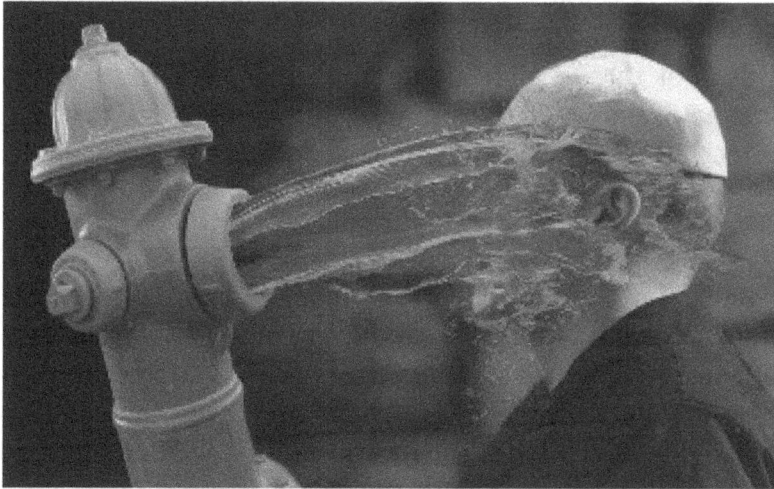

The slang phrase "drinking from a firehose" describes a common student complaint of the overwhelming feeling that classes in medical science usually engender. From the first day of classes, teachers blast you with massive amounts of information. This horrible feeling can happen whether the student is pursuing a career as a physician, dentist, medical researcher, nurse, or allied health professional. The sheer quantity of information in fields of medicine overwhelms the learner. Even a very thirsty person would still likely drown if trying to sip water from a gushing fire hose. Students in medical training may feel a similar terror of drowning. This book will focus on the tendency to "miss seeing the forest for the trees."

The quantity of information relevant to the delivery of health care never stops growing. New medications, new techniques, and new understandings keep coming. Every field of study grows in complexity over time, but medicine perhaps has an extra wrinkle. Since mastery of an enormous breadth of knowledge in medicine could impact a patient's chance of survival, the "firehose effect" seems especially ominous.

This book throws a lifeline to individuals pursuing a career in health care. If they expect and dread the "firehose effect," they need and deserve supportive encouragement.

Let's get started.

You do not have a standard textbook in your hands. This book does not pretend to espouse rigorous findings widely applicable. Instead, it contains observations from a clinician and his colleagues. The reader must judge if they make sense. The author has accumulated thousands of hours of healthcare experience, mostly spent in operating rooms. But still the reader should maintain a skeptical bias. Accept only those ideas that prove themselves compelling and useful.

Textbook authors never write in the first person, but I will. I will tell you stories from my own experiences. I think real experiences best convey concepts in a manner that sticks in the reader's mind. But bear in mind, similar situations do not always unfold to identical conclusions. In the final analysis, while we all use the experience of others as a guide to our lives, we each still maintain both the right and obligation to reach conclusions for ourselves.

I will share insights that I feel enhance learning. More importantly, I encourage students to search for consolidating, conceptual images for themselves even when their teacher fails to guide that vital step in mastery. That search requires a willingness to risk, to conjecture, and eventually to test one's suppositions. Eventually we will explore the choice of the word "**perspicacity**" in the title. Moving one's learning beyond the memorization of facts demands significant effort. I wish it were easy.

For many years the Walt Disney Company recognized America's best teachers with annual awards. In the 1980s, a television network carried one of their awards ceremonies. At that event, a winning science teacher explained that he taught courses three times to his students. In the first week, he covered the major concepts of the entire body of material. Next, he taught conventionally, point-by-point, over the semester. Finally, in the last two weeks, he summarized the complete course with an emphasis on how each idea contributed to the importance of the entire topic. That approach to teaching seemed novel and brilliant, and yet also self-evident once explained. As a student, have you experienced a teacher who taught you in that manner? Instead, most students seemingly must figure out on their own those first and last components of this idealized course structure. We want our teachers to help us understand the scope and insights of course material. But that commonly does not happen.

Our effort in writing Medical Investigation 101 brought into vivid focus the enormous range of elements we juggle in medical training. Medical science courses all share varying amounts of this tangle of dimensions. They all have a unique vocabulary, a history of the development of ideas, facts that one must memorize, and underlying concepts that pull together the lessons into useable skills. In addition, medicine has numerous tricky procedures requiring both manual and conceptual skills that practitioners must study and then practice to a high level of competence.

Consider this analogy. If you wish to learn to play the banjo, you need a little musical vocabulary and some understanding of notation, timing, and harmony. Additionally, you need hours upon hours practicing the manipulations required to make music blossom from that instrument.

The science of treating human disease and injury has thousands of unique words. Medicine has mountains of foundational science demanding mastery by those who render care. Medicine has procedures that require exhaustive practice. Procedural skills range from learning to differentiate the sounds captured by a stethoscope to honing the fine touch required to dissect one's way to an aneurysm inside the brain. *[We promise to define new words like aneurysm. An aneurysm looks like a widening or bulging artery. The bulge arises from a defect or injury in the wall of the artery. Over time the aneurysm can grow in size and eventually rupture. Sometimes an aneurysm produces symptoms, especially in the brain, by pushing on whatever structure lies close by.]*

Many career choices have multiple elements demanding mastery, even with levels of responsibility and dire consequences equivalent to medical practice. Such weighty obligations burden anyone pursuing such a demanding career. If you agree that teaching a course using the three-step teaching method has advantages, we should definitely use it for our most demanding professions. That does not happen routinely today. Medical courses typically do not start with a week of scope and vision for the material or end with a period of content integration. In the pages that follow, we are going to suggest insights into medical science courses that students might use as models for integrating the content of conventionally taught classes for themselves.

A critic might argue that the duty to formulate insights rightly belongs to the student and not the teacher. Perhaps, a critic might say, that step constitutes a crucial part of gaining competence in a field of study. That view has merit, but it appears that students still can earn degrees without formulating insights. Insights seem to have a visual quality, meaning one can "see" relationships and perhaps draw diagrams or maps to illustrate concepts. Humans appear to have remarkable abilities to formulate image analogues in their minds that enhance understanding. We can even manipulate these images to derive new perspectives. Exams rarely evaluate the students visual understanding of the course material.

A professor asked me an insightful question in a final oral examination for my doctorate in electrical engineering. He asked me to describe a visual model of the transformation of an electrical signal into the frequency domain as a path to determine its correlation with a reference signal. He asked me precisely that question. The question has relevance to the mathematics of electrical signal processing, but professors do not teach that concept visually. A painful effort ensued in my brain over many seconds, which felt like centuries. The professor listened to my crude effort to respond for a few minutes. Then, mercifully, he suggested I should work on that answer later. Fortunately, he passed me based, I hope, on a few better responses that I made during the examination.

Medical science differs greatly in its structure from engineering. *[A friend reviewed the draft of this book and suggested that I need to explain this observation in greater detail. My studies in engineering had a classic organization with individual classes consisting of about three hours of lecture each week. If I had 5 courses, I sat in class 15 hours not counting the possibility of some sort of lab experience. In graduate school I had a year in which I only worked on my thesis meeting once a week with my advisor for one hour. Teaching oneself represents a major allocation of time in such programs. Medical school represented a stark difference. For the first two years I sat with my classmates in a lecture hall for about seven hours a day, five days a week. I did not expect so much time spent sitting and listening. Many medical schools have specific courses in the same way one does in high school, while a growing number of schools are adopting an "organ-based curriculum." In the organ-based approach the first year goes through each major organ system one at a time including the anatomy, physiology, chemistry, and histology. The first year focuses on the normal, but the second year repeats the sequence with a focus on pathology. Organ systems would include musculoskeletal, respiratory, cardiovascular, endocrine, etc. Other medical science curricula for healthcare practitioners also seems to feature a great many hours of lecture.]*

Historically, medical therapies developed through inductive observation of treatments that seemed to work, cataloged over centuries. Understanding why came later, if ever. To this day, medical practitioners use remedies that appear to work even when we do not know how they work. But I want to urge students to focus at the beginning and throughout their careers on a search for foundational insights. That quest we are calling **perspicacity**. As we explore specific cases of reaching for the why, we will find that **perspicacity** may draw upon lessons from basic science, not from facts we have memorized from our medical training. Sometimes we get a new perspective just by imagining ourselves as a cell or a molecule, or even a gene. That may sound silly, but sometimes "silly" fosters revelation. We are going to explore.

Charles Darwin originated a notion of "hair splitters" vs. "lumpers" in a letter he wrote in 1857. Darwin noticed that he desired to know what various things have in common, more than he cared about how they differ. He called himself a lumper. Others instead seemed to dwell on details or "hair-splitting." You may have come across such divergent perspectives in yourself and others. "Splitters" appear to have comfort with a list of details. "Lumpers" beg to know the how and why. We want to advocate for lumping in this book. **Perspicacity** appears to favor the lumping philosophy.

"Lumpers" seek simplification. Albert Einstein once said, "If you can't explain it to a six-year-old, you don't understand it yourself." We are looking for insights. The word insight suggests a visual understanding, and we commonly find that a visual analogy makes it possible to explain a complicated idea even to a child. When we look for insights, keep in mind that we are seeking a visual understanding.

13

You may have the impression that Albert Einstein discovered secrets of physics that others could not understand by solving mathematical equations. Not true. It seems Einstein himself debunked that notion in his writings. Einstein studied experiments that produced observations that the current understanding of physics could not explain. He then opined, mused, or thought "what if" for many, many, many hours. You may have opined similarly, especially if you commonly awaken at 4 A.M. with great ideas.

Einstein kept at this questioning behavior with superhuman determination. He reported that in time he would find a visual analogy that appeared to explain an experimental riddle. In other words, the image that Einstein saw in his mind's eye unraveled the mysteries of physics. After seeing these visual solutions, he set about to describe his insight using the language of mathematics, often getting help with math from others. Seriously! The "insights" came from pictures in his mind, and mathematics came later. Remember that insight has a "visual" quality! This book, do I dare to say, hopes to create more Einstein-like students pursuing medical credentials.

We are entering an age in which we view the idea of learning in a fresh way. We see that artificial intelligence is taking over many of the skills that humans once uniquely embodied. As children we start school finding that learning requires the memorization of letters, numbers, colors, vocabulary, and even acceptable parameters of behavior. Teachers at that level spend most of their energy conducting "retrieval practice." In other words, they spend more time exercising memory function than presenting their students with new information.

Computers, by the way, surpassed humans at memorization from their inception. Something put into digital memory reliably stays put there indefinitely. More recently, computers took a step forward beyond memorization and programmed manipulations into "artificial intelligence." Humans have created computing machines that can figure out how to improve their capabilities through trial and error. The improvement in performance comes about through goal-based adjustments built into the machine's characteristics. Such computers have thus moved beyond carrying out a list of programmed manipulations. Instead, they can find methods to achieve a goal that never occurred to the programmer.

Goal-based processing starts out in a mode akin to how one might look for the top of a hill in the dark. A person could test with their toe in all directions to identify the direction of steepest ascent. Then take one step in that direction and test again. Stop when a step in every direction would move you downward. That technique leads you to the top of a hill. Other hills may rise higher. But a computer doing a process like the one we just described can be viewed as learning a path upward.

As an engineering student, my professor for a course called "Learning and Adaptive Machines," was consulting with the U.S. Post Office. He was helping them create machines that could learn how to read handwritten addresses on envelopes. The Post Office wanted machines to sort the mail. The post office had scanned thousands of envelopes and coded the correct interpretation of the address for each scan. The consulting engineers were using that collection of information as training materials to build a computer that could learn how to read handwritten addresses. The characteristics of each squiggle in the address had an associated probability of being a specific letter. The computer was learning its way to the hilltop of probabilities for each letter by the method we just described. Eventually the computer could use its map of hilltops it learned to decide what letter it was reading in a brand-new address. We were just starting back then to understand how computers could learn for themselves how to do a task. That process must have some relationship to the way children learn to tell a handwritten letter "m" from the letter "p."

Using our visual image of finding the path to the top of a hill in the dark, the next higher level of learning would add the ability to look beyond the next step to take in the dark. We want a method that can see more distant opportunities to find a global mountain top instead of merely a local hilltop. In the ultimate stage, humans and machines strive for learning that reflects back on the governing principles of reality to provide comprehension that can deduce an understanding we wish to achieve. That step mimics the process Einstein explained in his essay.

The element of shrewdness we find in the definition of **perspicacity** makes this word ideal to point us to the highest level of learning that we seek. In this book, we are asking how to promote perspicacious learning amidst the fire hose of information in medical science. A fire hose can readily put out the flame of **perspicacity**. It often does. We seek to make the student of medical science aware and alert to that possibility. And able to defend against it. Amidst a torrent of information to digest, we want to still ask how and why. A visual image of the underlying process endows us with **perspicacity**.

A classmate of mine in medical school developed a bulge in his wrist near the place where one commonly feels the radial pulse. We were just starting our second year of medical studies and were not acquainted with the concept of a ganglion cyst. The capsule that surrounds a joint between bones can sometimes develop a herniation, meaning a place that protrudes abnormally. In the case of a ganglion cyst, the joint space, by chance, develops an internal one-way-valve. The lubricating fluid inside the joint passes through the valve during regular movement, but cannot freely return. As a consequence, the captured liquid pushes the capsule outward, creating a bulge one can see and feel under the skin.

My classmate took his concern to the Student Health Office on campus. A very experienced physician examined the bothersome bump briefly and asked my comrade to excuse him for a moment while he fetched a book. Although we were still beginners in the study of medical science, we knew that physicians did not routinely go looking for a book during the examination of a patient. Needing to consult a textbook might erode a patient's confidence in their physician. While personally experiencing the "fire-hose effect," my classmate suddenly felt awe for this experienced physician who had the self-confidence to consult a book right in front of his patient. As he waited for the doctor to return, he was thinking warmly about this turn of events. Perhaps he too could consult a book when his memory failed him when he assumed the role of the physician. Indeed, this idea seemed comforting to him as he waited for the doctor's return.

In a few minutes, the practitioner returned with an enormous book. By then, my classmate was looking forward to the process of consulting the book with the doctor. Indeed, he was considering talking to him about his worries about memorizing everything he would need to know in his future career. Instead, without warning, this experienced physician slammed the heavy book down squarely on his patient's wrist, still outstretched on the examination table. The blow ruptured the ganglion cyst at the same time that it ended his philosophical musing. We laughed when our comrade told us this harrowing story, but our laughter had a sympathetic, painful quality. We secretly shared his concern that our ability to memorize might eventually fail us. We needed a rescue strategy. Is there a different approach to the mastery of medical science?

We all were hoping the book in this story was going to be used differently.

[*Commonly, the definitive treatment of a ganglion cyst requires surgical removal of the "one-way valve" inside the joint space. In the lore of medical practice of bygone eras, the general practitioner may have kept a hefty Bible in the office to rupture ganglion cysts. Many ruptured cysts recurred. Apparently, surprise significantly enhanced the efficacy of this therapy as taught back then. Probably patients with a recurrence were less cooperative with a violent whopping with the "Good Book."*]

Chapter 2: Barriers to Medical Education

Medical careers oft hit two grave barricades,
Fainting at blood and yucky O-Chem grades.
The O-Chem torture one must grimly endure,
But the fainting concern I can quickly cure.

Before diving into **perspicacity**, I want to complain vehemently that far too many highly qualified students have crossed medical studies off their list of possible careers. They did so because of Organic Chemistry or because the sight of blood makes them faint. We need to face up to these two issues! We need to confront them honestly and definitively!

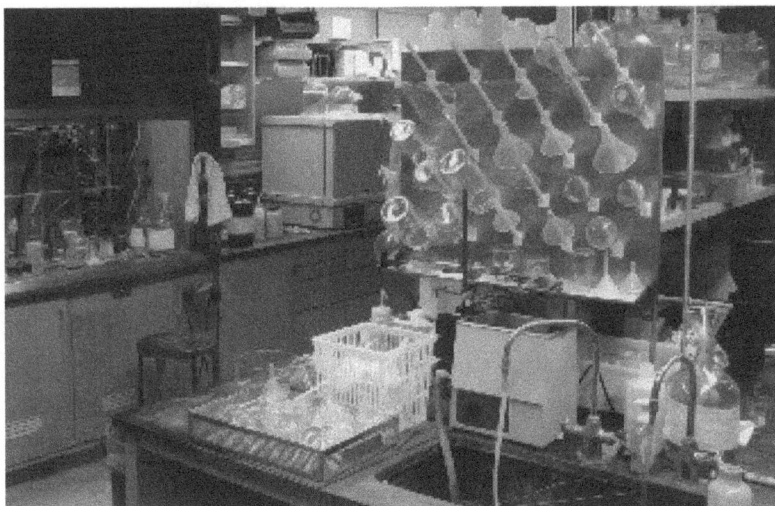

Organic Chemistry has earned a horrible reputation, probably with valid reasons. Like medical science courses, the traditional Organic Chemistry class rapidly overwhelms the student with a zillion bizarre molecule names and structures that prove hellacious to memorize. In some universities, the laboratory experience for this class may not match-up with the lecture, and that can further disorient the diligent student. Over the years, medical schools have required Organic Chemistry as a prerequisite primarily to weed-out students who might lack the grit needed to complete medical school studies. It probably does that, but it likely also robs our society of some wonderfully caring medical practitioners.

I confess that I have no secret for rendering Organic Chemistry easy. The course does demand fortitude. Try to take Organic Chemistry during a lighter workload semester and budget bountiful study time for this class. Learning some Organic Chemistry vocabulary and playing with three-dimensional models of the standard organic molecules before starting the course can make the experience less overwhelming. Once the course begins, work at it diligently every day. I wish I had more to offer. Expect a grind and stick with it.

Now move along to the queasy stomach problem. Everyone who ever considered a career in healthcare has had the concern that confronting "blood and guts" might render them dysfunctional, one way or another. The popularity of the British television comedy "Doc Martin" only adds to such a concern. The show portrays a fictional surgeon forced by the fear of seeing blood to stop doing surgery. The concept seems reasonable, except that it only happens in fiction. The reason deserves an explanation.

We can all imagine the possibility that a gory spectacle might deposit us fainted in a heap upon the floor at the very moment that we want to display powerful composure and poise. You might imagine that no one but you have that concern. In fact, everyone has that worry! Still, you can forget about it. Seriously, you can completely forget about that concern! Please read that last sentence again to yourself slowly in your most convincing inner tone of voice.

Here's what actually happens. During your medical training, you will come upon perhaps a hundred lessons you want never to forget. You appreciate that a patient in acute distress one day will need you to know what to do to save their life. You will study all these lessons because you know their importance. Then, one day, when you least expect it, an honest-to-God gory situation will present itself. At that moment, you will go into overdrive doing everything you have learned how to do to save a life. It will not occur to you that gore surrounds you. Hours later, you might recall that you stood elbow deep in overwhelming carnage.

You might never realize that you entirely ignored such gruesome gore. So, forget about fainting or any embarrassing reactions to gory events. Spectators have those reactions, not people who have a responsible, complicated job to perform. When the time comes, you are going to act expertly, even if you do not believe me at this moment. It happens absolutely that way.

If you are determined to pursue a career in healthcare, these two hurdles should never stand in your way. Now let's move on to more crucial insights.

Chapter 3: The Chemistry of Life

You find Bunsen burners on every chemistry bench,
Cause it takes really high heat to make atoms unclench.
But life depends on atoms rearranging,
Rearranging to keep our bodies changing.
How can this happen way down at 98 degrees?
That's a big issue for bees, fleas, trees, knees, and me(s).

So how does all of the chemistry of life happen at room temperature? Why do chemists need Bunsen burners to carry out chemical reactions in the laboratory?

Our bodies break apart the molecules in our food and rearrange atoms into brand new materials without needing Bunsen burners. Without any high heat, our bodies perform chemistry for energy, for growing, and for repairing worn out parts. The answer to this puzzle constitutes perhaps the essential secret of life. It goes to the core of how life emerged from this sphere of once molten rock we humans call the planet earth.

When we hold a plastic cup in our hands, we grasp a material made of large, long molecules. I mean large and long compared to most other molecules. Molecules consist of atoms that fit together in a specific pattern. Indeed, it takes considerable energy (heat) to pull those atoms apart once they have joined together into a stable chemical compound.

Imagine collecting a pile of rocks, each with a different shape and size. If you push them all together, you still simply have a collection of stones. But instead, view these rocks as pieces of a puzzle that you might carefully fit together to form a stone wall. Tourists in Connecticut admire the abundance of such stone walls, built in years gone by without mortar. Stones snuggly fitted together can stand strong and tall for centuries. Atoms act similarly, except when introduced into molecules they initially resist. When forced, they can pop firmly into place to create a new stable compound. The heat from a Bunsen burner in the chemistry laboratory does that "forcing."

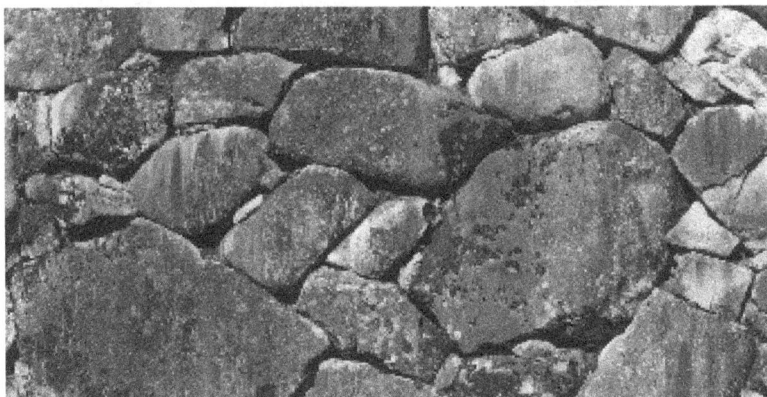

Inside our body, we coax atoms into molecules using enzymes. Enzymes substitute for high heat. An enzyme, itself a protein molecule, consists of various atoms fitted together, like our analogy of a stone wall, built upon a skeleton of carbon atoms. Remember, the dictionary defines Organic Chemistry as the chemistry of carbon-based molecules. Biologists would say life, as we know it, relies upon carbon atoms. Life, as we know it, depends upon the miracle of enzymes.

As an aside, the physicist Enrico Fermi, famous for creating the first controlled nuclear reactor under Stagg Field in Chicago in 1942, also originated the "Fermi Paradox." The

Fermi Paradox suggests that life must exist elsewhere in the universe because of the vast number of planets available out yonder upon which life could emerge. On the other hand, if life only exists on the planet earth, we might blame that on the vastly low probability of randomly creating the miracle of the enzyme. Philosophers have suggested that enough monkeys typing randomly on keyboards would eventually reproduce the works of Shakespeare. That outcome would take a very long time. Getting back to enzymes, creating the first enzyme, definitely took a long while to happen if it arose from random events. You might say that humans essentially won the lottery just to be alive.

Atoms have a nucleus surrounded by a cloud of orbiting electrons. Since electrons have a negative charge that repels other electrons, electrons prefer to stay away from each other. This cloud of electrons creates resistance for atoms trying to move tightly together. The electron cloud also creates a resistance to attempting to pull atoms out of a molecule once they have fitted tightly together. You can picture this effect in your mind. The electrons happily orbiting a single nucleus have a stable status.

The electrons belonging, indeed surrounding each atom, resist being pushed close to other atoms also surrounded by electrons. But if pushed hard enough, the electron clouds can potentially meld together.

Then all of the electrons can again find happiness orbiting about the entire new molecule. That ability to blend does not exist for all combinations of atoms. But if they can meld into a happier arrangement, the electrons then resist any attempt to pull the molecule apart. (You will recognize that

I have used happiness to mean a lower energy state. I hope I have not insulted any readers with this liberal analogy.)

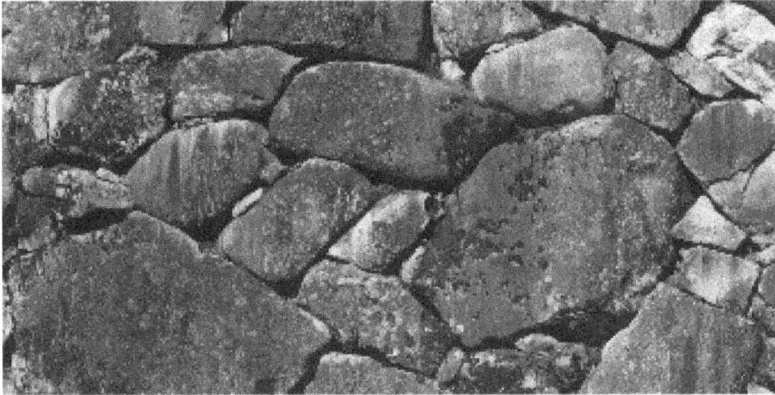

Now, suppose an enzyme comes along. The enzyme acts like a scaffold that fits precisely around specific atoms and molecules. It seemingly distracts the orbiting electrons and allows the atoms to all come together readily to form a new molecule. The enzyme dissipates that initial resistance to blending the electron clouds. Next, the enzyme breaks away, making the enzyme again available to do its magic trick to form other atoms into a copy of that same new molecule. Life requires many different enzymes. These various enzymes bring about virtually all the essential chemical reactions that take place inside our bodies. Enzymes work away inside all forms of life, as we know it, enabling chemical reactions without a Bunsen burner. It's magic that works away silently all around and inside of us. We should regard the human body as a very talented chemical factory employing in the range of 75,000 different enzymes that carry out the necessary assembly and disassembly of compounds we need to live. The cells of our body stay very busy.

To appreciate the miracle of the enzyme more thoroughly, we need to ask why humans go to the trouble of regulating our body temperature to 98.6 degrees Fahrenheit. Temperature describes the energy of movement, perhaps better described as vibration, of atoms and molecules. On a hot day, molecules and atoms that make up the atmosphere are zinging about energetically, banging into each other. They also slam into us and transfer some of their energy to us, causing us to feel hot. When atoms and molecules vibrate about with increased energy, they tend to want more space.

We see this effect when warming expands the fluid inside a glass thermometer, demonstrating visually how warm the day has become. Enzymes also alter their size as the temperature changes. We have learned that the usefulness of the enzyme depends upon its ability to fit precisely around specific groupings of atoms and meld their electron clouds. Therefore, we can appreciate that a temperature change could alter the enzyme's capability. Enzymes inside our body appear to work best at 98.6 degrees Fahrenheit, so evolution favored keeping our body at that temperature. Some life forms lack that temperature regulation ability. When it gets cold, trees do not grow, and humans get a rest from mowing their grass. Reptiles and amphibians do not regulate their body's temperature, so they become dormant when the ambient temperature drops. Some of these species have the ability to increase the glucose level in their bloodstream to lower the freezing point of their circulation.

Later, we will consider why germs manufacture molecules called pyrogens that cause human temperature regulation to malfunction, giving us a fever. Many of our insights into medical science involve stepping back to ask why. Why would evolution favor a particular aspect of human physiology? Darwin taught mankind the idea of evolution as a formative process in nature. That concept serves as a foundational basis for many medical insights. The processes by which the human body achieves its goals, we call physiology. The ways the human body can falter in its performance we call pathology. We might say that pathology is to illness as physiology is to health. In this book, we will often ask why evolution would favor some odd way our body goes about solving a problem. Asking that question takes us beyond regurgitating a memorized answer on an examination. By asking why, we seek to uncover an insight that will enhance our understanding and expand our quest to improve health care.

Shall we keep going?

Chapter 4 The Miracle of Coagulation

When something happens that causes one to bleed,
We need to stop the bleeding at full warp speed.
So how would you design a counter measure,
To reliably protect this life, we treasure.

Back in 1960, comedian Bob Newhart recorded a record album that won him a Grammy Award. On that album, he pretended, as an agent of manufacturer Olympic Games Inc., to take a telephone call from Abner Doubleday wanting to promote his invention that he called baseball. The humor of the skit lies in hearing someone try to explain the complexity of baseball in a phone call. Who could possibly think a game so convoluted in its rules could prove successful?

Now suppose you were to study the biochemistry of blood coagulation. That topic makes Doubleday's game seem simple. Baseball has 18 players, but forming a clot to stop bleeding, has 20 players. The coagulation players are called Clotting Factors, and they all have uniform numbers (one through twenty). They have names like Protein C, Antithrombin III, Christmas Factor, and Proaccelerin.

Apparently, Factor 6 got traded to another team, so it merely has an empty space on the roster. Like baseball, we have two sides, the Extrinsic and the Intrinsic Teams. Recently, it seems members of the "Intrinsics" have been cheating by helping out the Extrinsic Team. I am not making this up.

Students of medical science typically find the study of coagulation arduous. They live through it and memorize enough details to pass the examination, but they rarely phone their Moms to share their excitement over this experience.

Why does coagulation need so much complexity? It took years for scientific research and many investigators to put all of the details together. Edits and corrections still pop up in the literature.

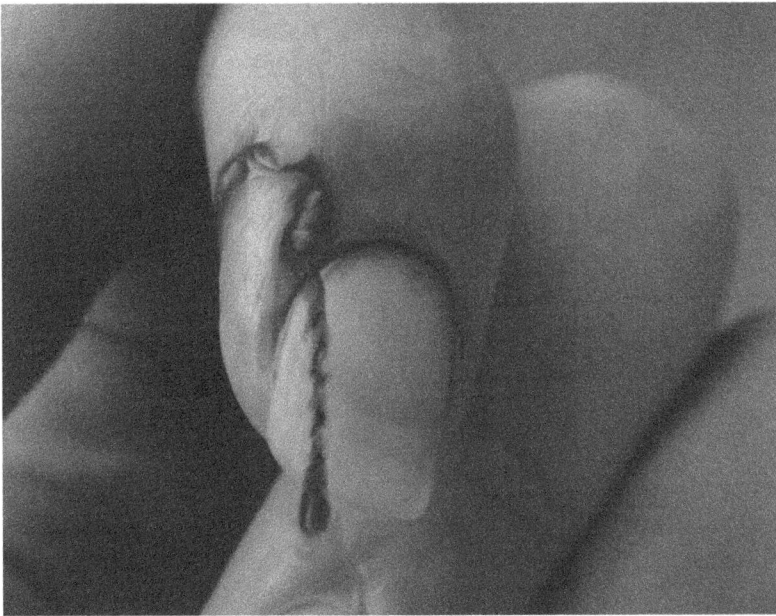

Why would evolution want to have 19 different components required just to make a clot? I know earlier I said twenty factors, but remember, number 6 bowed out.

Should every publication on this topic begin by explaining why coagulation needs so much complexity? Of course! Yet, I cannot find a single article that addresses that issue at all. Instead, experts create diagrams and lists to explain how all of these relationships interact. They use arrows to show how factors activate one another. Still, as best I can find, they never say why it needs such an elaborate procedure.

Does the complexity of coagulation need no explanation because it seems obvious to everyone but me? In preparation for writing this chapter, I asked some of my friends in medical science, "Why is coagulation so complicated?" They commonly repeated my question to make sure I really asked them such a silly question. Then they said something like, "It's complicated because it needs to be." I countered vigorously, "It needs to work reliably, so it should have simplicity."

I want to suggest an alternative answer to my question. Forming a clot has two key, irksome challenges that the design must accomplish. First, coagulation must amplify a very subtle stimulus into millions of chemical reactions to form clots within seconds to successfully stop bleeding. Second, the process cannot permit clotting to go wild and clot everything.

I would start a lecture on coagulation with a discussion of those two design criteria. A few minutes spent thinking hard about those two objectives, I believe, would make the topic of clot formation much more exciting. What does it take to achieve those two objectives, and how did biology solve this dilemma?

First, what do we know concerning speed? In economics, scholars talk about the miracle of compound interest in making money quickly. Engineers lump issues of speed under the umbrella of "gain" or amplification. A bleed allows a few molecules of tissue from the outside of the vessel to come in contact with blood. The presence of these few molecules that usually would never touch flowing blood initiates the clotting when a vessel ruptures. Our body must amplify the influence of a few molecules a lot.

A single-stage activation sequence cannot get that job done quickly. We need multiple layers of doubling and tripling. We should, therefore, expect to see one substance activate another substance, and that, in turn, activate another. Each activation stage multiplies the previous step, and strings of multiplication increase exponentially. Exponential growth makes a critical difference in speed. We should expect to find chains of multiplication in the diagrams of coagulation. And we do, but physiologists do not add labels that say, "exponential growth stages."

Our second objective requires that we keep coagulation from running amuck. Scientists label this process fibrinolysis. Textbooks say that congenital disorders in fibrinolysis occur rarely. Of course, a fetus with a defect in fibrinolysis would rarely survive to be born. Electrical engineers take classes to learn how to design control systems that work with precision and stability. Gain, as we mentioned, constitutes an essential ingredient of such control systems.

So, we should expect a biochemical process to have multiple stages of activation to provide its gain. Sure enough, we find activators and enzymes triggering and inhibiting one another in the fibrinolytic system.

Students still need to memorize lots of names and relationships to pass their exams. Yet an image of the way an oven heats to a specific controlled temperature and then hold at the set point might make the lesson more engaging.

31

Nature solved these engineering problems through evolution, while humans use mathematics and slide rules.

Chapter 5 Why do germs and viruses hate us?

Germs and viruses go about making folks ill,
Don't you wonder if they have any other skill?
Their raison d'etre lacks even an iota of glee,
If they leave me alone, I would surely let them be.

My infectious disease class ranks as the absolute worst class in my medical school curriculum. Decades later, I still rue the fact that I wasted so much time in that class, never learning what I wanted to know. For eight weeks, we had one lecture each hour of the school day, each on a different disease.

Every infectious disease seemed to cause malaise and fever. "Malaise" was not part of my vocabulary before taking this course. I knew it meant some vague feeling of sickness. The course gave me "malaise."   After eight weeks of this regimen, I had no idea how to begin to figure out what was causing any specific patient's malaise and fever. I hoped that a culture of some bodily fluid would yield the diagnosis. I also hoped a lab test for drug sensitivity would tell me what drug might help the patient, since otherwise I had no clue. I felt that I had wasted 8 weeks of my life. I kept asking myself, "How could a brilliant professor at a reputable medical school decide this was the way to teach future physicians how to manage infectious diseases." To this day, the organization of that course makes no sense to me at all.

My classmates and I needed a "lumper" in charge instead of a "splitter."

From that horrible beginning, it seems ironic that I would want to put a chapter in this book of insights devoted to infectious disease. But I do.

I am doing so just in case other medical schools might still teach this material in this same frustrating manner. The medical literature clearly suggests a profound change in perspective on germs and viruses has come about over the last several decades. That change may have replaced the fever and malaise lecture series with some much more exciting insights into this crucial topic in healthcare.

I really hope so!

In my medical school years, too many years ago, the axiom "the only good germ is a dead one" held sway. Hospitals back then, and many still today, wash every possible surface at least daily with potent toxic fluids designed to kill everything tiny. Despite that practice, patients do pick up new infections in hospitals. I classify these hospital infections as "doozies" because these "doozy" germs have survived the lethal fluids modern science designed to kill them. And these "doozy" germs also tend to evade the lethality of the antibiotics hospitals then infuse into patients made ill by these microbes.

Massacring germs may not prove the ideal strategy for protecting hospital patients. Does any other approach exist? A few parts of the world have used cow manure as a poultice for wounds, not something we find in industrialized nations. How might this manure strategy work? Manure teems with bacteria. But the bacteria in manure comes from the digestive-track of cattle and almost entirely falls in the category of non-pathogenic bacteria (bacteria that do not cause disease). Filling a wound with

34

non-pathogenic bacteria makes it very difficult for pathogenic bacteria to gain a foothold. The dangerous bacteria in this situation have too much competition even to get noticed. I cannot find any hospitals near me that actively introduce non-pathogenic bacteria into their patient care units to compete with the pathogens they want to suppress.

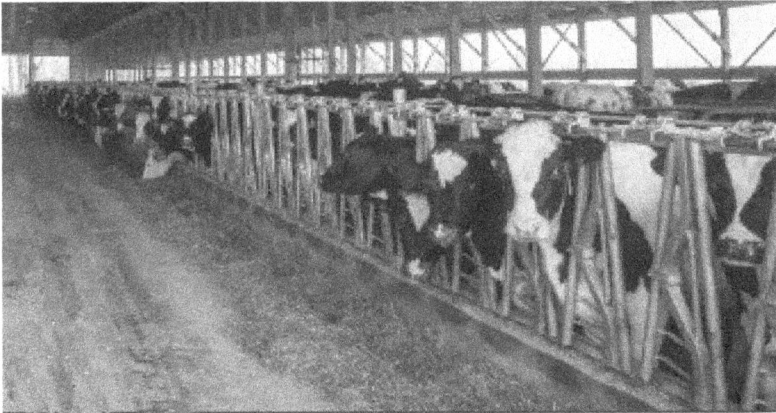

You may recall that Joseph Lister advocated handwashing in the 1860s as the primary remedy for the hospital-acquired infection problem. Unfortunately, this problem remains today. Might we need to mimic the cow manure approach? Is there a more esthetically acceptable variation on this approach?

Let's look around for an idea. The manufacture of alcoholic beverages requires fermentation. Fermentation means that living microbes, yeast, use their enzyme skills to change sugars found in grapes and other fruits and grains into alcohol. These talented yeast varieties also crank out esters that give our favorite brews their distinctive and alluring tastes. Hundreds of different species of yeast have been identified. Each one seems to have its own distinct set of enzymes that determine the final taste of the beverage. Vineyards, brewers, and distillers all want to deliver for their customers precisely the same beverage taste year after year. That objective proves quite tricky. Consistency requires that the fermenting microbes and growing conditions of the raw materials all stay the same. Strict sterility might seem the best strategy for maintaining consistency in the fermentation part of the process. However, some processors instead borrow a plan from the "manure wound care approach." They paint their entire facility with the microbes they prefer, electing the "manure" strategy over the "sterile" strategy.

To keep from falling victim to infectious diseases, we can either kill all the microbes or perhaps dilute them with harmless germs. But why have human beings not merely evolved immunity to all bacteria and viruses?

Human beings evolved so many extraordinary skills, how did we fail at this one? The tiniest forms of biological life appear to have a unique evolutionary advantage. The trick comes from something straightforward and basic. Since evolution improves genetic traits through inheritance, organisms with short generation spans evolve faster. The generation span for humans ranges from 22 to 33 years. For germs, a generation span ranges from 12 minutes to 14 hours (depending heavily on the ambient temperature for life forms that cannot control their body temperature). So, we should expect germs to evolve more than 8000 times faster than humans. For that simple reason, the saber tooth tiger has become much less dangerous to humans over time than the more rapidly evolving pathogenic bacteria and viruses.

I did learn in medical school that whenever a febrile patient with malaise has traveled recently to a developing nation, they need a PPD. A PPD test (purified protein derivative or a Mantoux test) shows if the patient has ever been exposed to tuberculosis (TB). About 25% of the world's population has been exposed to tuberculosis, and about 10 million people fall seriously ill from this life-threatening disease each year. A skin test for tuberculosis makes sense for patients living in America. On the other hand, this test has little value in nations where TB occurs commonly. In those nations, almost everyone tests positive for having been exposed to the disease. Many people are exposed to tuberculosis without developing the disease.

Every year public health workers worldwide struggle to eradicate TB, so far without success. The short generation time of the tuberculosis bacterium appears to keep it one step ahead of our best efforts. The microbe evolves a new way to survive every new drug we create to rid it from the planet.

Recently we have begun to understand that bacteria serve us all as a natural, necessary part of our human physiology. We recognized many years ago that we require bacteria in our digestive system.

Bacteria help us break down the food we eat into simpler molecules that we can readily absorb and utilize. More recently, we have found that bacteria live in other parts of our body and assist our physiology in ways we are just beginning to comprehend. Researchers at the National Institutes of Medicine near Washington, D.C., have found that adding different bacteria into the colon of patients can treat many conditions, even emotional disorders. That's a big surprise. Findings like that suggest we have much to learn about how our body interacts with bacteria and viruses.

We could benefit from new insights into our relationship with these tiny organisms that affect our lives. Viruses, unlike bacteria, are technically not alive. A virus consists of only a snippet of genetic material wrapped up in a protein capsule. Unlike living microbes, a virus cannot reproduce without help. A virus must invade a living cell to reproduce itself.

The cell contributes the apparatus to duplicate the virus's genetic material and manufacture the protein needed for the viral coat. We might start a search for a deeper understanding by asking, "How did the first virus come into existence?" A virus obviously could not exist before there were other cell-based forms of life. "Why would a cell create that first virus?"

In our minds, the temptation exists to assume that the first virus arose from some evil intent. Evil intent seems such a sophisticated concept that it probably did not exist when the first virus appeared on earth.

Indeed, plant biologists have discovered that viruses found on plants can help the plant survive droughts and other adverse natural conditions. This finding suggests that a virus perhaps may act as an "outsourced trait or skill. " By "outsourced," I mean that the plant created the virus to store a snippet of DNA that gives the plant a valuable survival trait. Instead of storing this skill encoded among the plant's other genomes, it put it on a "shelf" outside of itself. Saving a capability in this manner might benefit the plant by requiring less expenditure of energy to maintain or perpetuate the skill. We find these viruses on the surface of the plant and inside the seeds of the plant.

I find this discovery fascinating. This discovery may lead scientists to many more crucial insights. Could it prove possible that human beings also utilize a viral strategy to store genetic skills? Might a virus that causes a human illness have started as an outsourced trait of a plant or other animal, or even a human?

The concept of evolution tells us that entities that persist and evolve in nature must exhibit some improvement or advantage. When we ask, why do viruses exist, we have to look for a survival advantage that they create. Does a flu virus or a coronavirus create some improvement elsewhere in nature? We focus on the fact that it kills a significant number of humans. If it exists only to kill its host, we would not predict the prosperous future many viruses seem to enjoy. Possibly, if we fully understood the path of its evolution, we might recognize new ways to stop epidemics and pandemics. Of note, experts believe one of the flu pandemics in our history came from a virus created by humans in an Asian biological warfare laboratory. That intent would definitely appear sinister, but other viral agents might arise in nature without any evil purpose.

If you should elect to research this topic in the current medical literature, you can find fascinating observations. Seemingly these observations have not led to especially useful insights.

Suppose you were to create a new virus that had no purpose except to infect cells and reproduce a few copies of itself. If you painted the walls inside your house with this do-nothing virus, would it compete with viruses that cause illness? That might provide a benefit to humans. But it also might prove harmful by diluting out viruses that aid human beings, viral outsourced human traits that we currently do not appreciate.

The world as close as our own skin may have friends and enemies that we poorly understand at present. Perhaps we can create viruses that serve as vaccinations and spread disease immunity instead of disease.

This book contains another chapter that discusses the virus in a different context. We could put that chapter next, but some benefit may derive from postponing it until you have read other examples of **perspicacity** to shape your thinking. Medical science has barely begun in its comprehension of the virus.

Chapter 6 Cancer

As a general rule of thumb,
Seek the very, very best outcome.
If cancer attacks your liver or heart,
Taking poison may not prove so smart.

Cancer appropriately ranks in the "top ten" of things people dread. We use words to describe this condition like deadly, insidious, unfair, relentless, incurable. Medical science appears to have stumbled in its fight against cancer when compared to progress in other areas. We know that cancer arises from alterations in the genetic instructions inside cells that allow those cells to reproduce aggressively. Cancerous cells fail to attach tightly to neighboring cells in the way typical cells bond. The lack of attachment allows cancerous cells to move about the body, a behavior referred to as metastasizing. We have searched diligently for "the" cause of cancer and found "many" possibilities.

As a society, we have acted to outlaw agents that have the potential to induce mutations in cells that lead to cancer. We call such agents carcinogens. On the list of known carcinogens, we find chemotherapeutic drugs and ionizing radiation. We still use both of these carcinogens to treat cancer. Epidemiological studies over the years have demonstrated that healthcare practitioners who treat cancer patients with these agents themselves have an elevated risk of developing cancer.

We might declare a medical science insight here. "Treating cancer with a therapy known to cause cancer cannot serve as the ultimate cure for cancer." That insight has not gone unnoticed by many inside and outside the ranks of medical practice. Still, the use of these modes of treatment has persisted. Fortunately, other options are coming along.

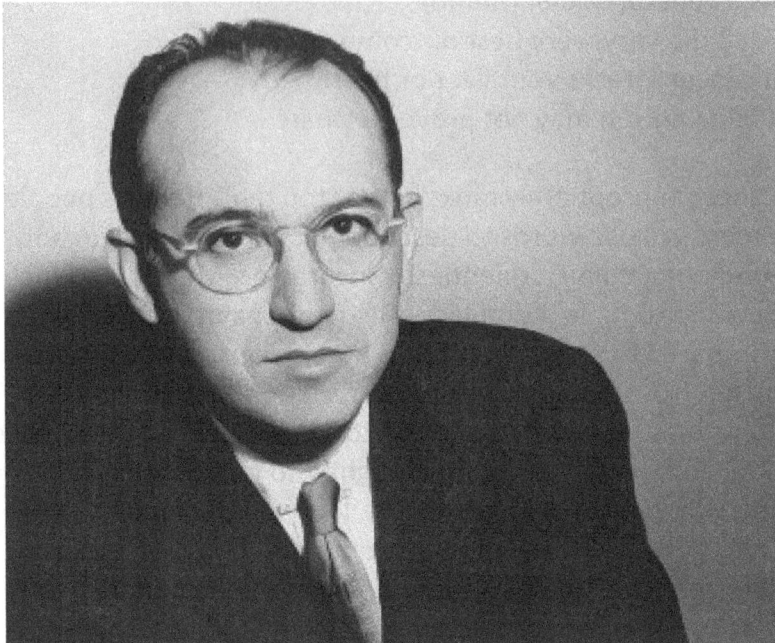

Jonas Salk (famous for his research that ended the polio plague) argued that we should not search for the causes of cancer. Instead, he urged scientists to figure out why everyone <u>does not</u> have cancer. Salk recognized that cells constantly mutate inside every human. The process of living requires the creation of new cells. Mistakes occur in the process of copying our genetic codes needed to create new cells to grow and repair ourselves.

Mistakes occur rarely. But the code elements copied in every cell division number in the billions. The number of cell divisions in our body each day reaches another huge number (probably unknowable). Some mistakes in copying genes inside cells can get corrected. Other errors can trigger white cells in our bloodstream to destroy the malfunctioning cells.

Currently, an exciting frontier of cancer research lies in improved gene mistake correction and better targeting of white cells to attack cancers.

These treatment approaches match the strategic advice Jonas Salk gave us many decades ago. The Salk advice provides a testimony to the power of seeking insights in medical science. Salk's idea takes us beyond merely exploiting the observation that carcinogenic agents can sometimes slow the progress of cancer. Oncologists (specialists in the treatment of cancer) would say that radiation and chemotherapy can put some patients into remission from their cancer. At the end of remission, we say the patient has suffered a recurrence. Commonly the recurrence of cancer no longer responds to the treatment that previously created that respite.

The pattern of remission followed by a more resistant cancer recurrence appears similar to the selection process of evolution. The therapy selects out the most resistance cancer cells to survive and eventually they return with the ability to resist the previously effective treatment.

This perspective makes the non-carcinogenic treatments that Dr. Salk hoped for much more appealing.

The conventional dosing strategy for radiation and chemotherapy seeks the destruction of all the cancerous cells in the patient. At least one cancer researcher asked what would happen if chemotherapy was dosed only to stop the growth of malignant tumors (not reduce their size). Animal studies of this strategy resulted in laboratory animals fighting off their induced cancer using their own white cells once the tumor growth halted. Oncologists have not widely adopted this strategy in human cancer therapy. The new gene- and immuno-based cancer treatments appear more promising. They would seem to deserve all the research attention we can afford them.

Chapter 7 Control Systems

If normal humans have a consistent finding,
It can't just arise from random combining.
A mechanism must exist to make that occur.
It takes a mechanism to ensure that norms concur.

When I began to study electrical engineering, I was surprised to find that many of my courses centered on control systems. Honestly, when I decided on graduate studies in electrical engineering, I had never considered that control systems would belong there. If asked to name a control system, I might have suggested a thermostat. I knew a wall-mounted thermostat fires up the furnace on a cold day. It keeps the furnace running until the room temperature rises to the desired warmth. At that point, the thermostat turns the furnace off. That notion would not seem to warrant a great deal of attention in a graduate program in engineering. Actually, I ended up studying control systems for a couple years.

The standard home thermostat does not represent a particularly fine control system. A room's temperature controlled by a standard thermostat does not stay precisely at the value one sets. The temperature climbs higher than the set temperature because the furnace does not immediately stop delivering heat the instant the thermostat turns off. Furthermore, the furnace does not start up again until the room temperature falls below the set temperature, usually by about a degree. The standard thermostat works precisely enough for our needs in home heating, but society needs much better control systems in many other applications.

If you wish to stop your automobile at an intersection where pedestrians cross, you would not want to depend upon a thermostat-like control. To stop an automobile, you want to control the position of the car more precisely by controlling both velocity and acceleration (deceleration in this case).

Fortunately, the human brain seems to have evolved an instinctive expertise for managing the physics of various objects sitting about our planet. Humans can capably control an automobile and bring it to a stop reliably at the edge of a crosswalk. Drivers do this task by letting up on the accelerator ahead of arrival and then by applying the brake expertly to bring the deceleration and the velocity of the vehicle both down to zero at the designated spot. Humans are more sophisticated controllers than thermostats that bang fully on and then bang fully off. Engineers literally refer to the thermostat as a "bang-bang" controller. They refer to the process humans use to stop a car as a proportional controller, meaning the adjustment of the controls has a proportional relationship to the error. By error they mean the difference between the current location of the automobile and the desired stopping point.

In healthcare we commonly evaluate patients by doing various tests that all have so-called normal values. If a test results in a finding that lies outside of the normal range of these measurements, we ask ourselves what caused that abnormality. An important medical insight is hiding here!

The key medical insight lies in recognizing that every normal value has an associated physiological control system. It takes special effort to keep a physiological measurement always at a specific level. Normal values do not appear in the human body by chance or coincidence. For example, a control system exists to make the normal value of potassium in the blood stay at the "normal value" for potassium concentration in the blood serum. An abnormal value suggests that either the control system has failed, or some circumstance has overwhelmed the ability of the control system to maintain that normal value. The healthcare provider then tries to figure out which of those possibilities has occurred, usually by adding in other observations or doing more lab tests to identify the diagnosis.

Most healthcare professionals have not studied the mathematics that engineers use to guide the design of a stable control system. But they do know how to stop their car reliably an arm's length from the fast-food drive-up window. That works very well for them. But I want you to recognize that a control system exists for every consistent feature in the human body. In some cases, no one may have yet figured out how that system works. Why is your left arm pretty much the same length as your right one? What sort of controller makes that happen? Have physiologists figured that out? Do we have a counting mechanism in our genetic coding that counts cell divisions to make each arm grow the same amount? I challenge you to think of questions to ask yourself about how our body controls processes as you think of traits that we find consistent among humans. Most people have ten toes, so we have a mechanism to control that. A few rare individuals have extra digits, suggesting something went astray with that mechanism.

When I started my residency training in anesthesiology after completing medical school, one of my clinical professors said, "Watch out for red heads." I thought at first that she was giving me dating advice. No, she was seriously telling me that patients with red hair frequently have unusual reactions to anesthetic medications, and one needs to be cautious. The anesthetist must very carefully titrate doses when taking care of these patients. [*Titrate might represent a new word for you. In medicine it simply means one monitors the patient continuously while giving small doses until the desired result appears.*] My professor was sharing a commonly understood admonition among anesthetists that I needed to follow. She did not tell me why red hair caused a sensitivity to anesthetics, although I think I asked for the reason.

Much later I learned that the chemicals that nerve cells use to communicate in the brain are synthesized in the same series of chemical reactions inside our body that create the pigment called melanin. When a person has red hair, they have a difference in their level of this pigment. But that means there likely are differences in other products made in that same chain of chemical reactions. Many red headed patients react with an unexpected sensitivity to one or more drugs used in the delivery of a general anesthetic.

Soon thereafter I had a red headed patient. I quizzed her very carefully about whether or not she had experienced any previous problem with medications or with anesthetics. She became suspicious of me and wanted to know if I always asked so many questions like that. I explained to her my concern was based on her hair color, and she told me I could relax because that color came from a bottle. She said she did appreciate my extensive efforts to keep her safe.

I want to take this medical insight a step further. In medical education students commonly learn specific doses for medications they might prescribe. A routine dose might read 200 milligrams taken three times a day. Another medication may have a recommendation for 4 milligrams daily per each kilogram of the patient's body weight. Potent medications with serious side effects might not be safely dosed using that sort of recipe.

Medications given to patients through an intravenous route (directly into a vein) usually work quickly and might be given in small doses until the patient exhibits the desired response. When medications are given in this fashion, we call that process "titration." Titrating a medication turns the medical practitioner into a control system. When students in health care first try to titrate medications for an actual patient, they tend to act just like a thermostat. They give a little dose, then another little dose, and they keep doing that until they get the patient to the desired objective. Suppose we use the objective of a systolic blood pressure of 110 millimeters of mercury for a patient who has fainted with a blood pressure of 70. After giving several small doses of neostigmine you read 110 and you stop giving doses. Next, you panic as the patient's blood pressure climbs to 160. What happened? Does your understanding of control systems allow you to recognize the problem? Of course. One needs to act like a proportional controller and give smaller doses as we get close to the objective, and perhaps give those doses further apart in time.

Engineers create a mathematical model of the way a process behaves when they set about to design a control system for a specific application. In the real world, the engineer may not know enough about the process behavior to do that, just as we cannot always predict a patient's reaction to a medication. How do engineers handle this problem of controlling a system that may change its behavior?

Consider an example. High performance military aircraft change their flight dynamics with changes in air temperature, air density, distribution of weight inside the plane, and changes in the fuel tanks' weight as fuel is used up. These variables significantly change the sensitivity of the plane responding to the pilot's hand movements on the controls during a flight. The engineers who designed the plane cannot know these factors ahead of time, and pilots may not be able to accurately adapt to the changes as they focus on a combat mission. The Air Force wants the pilot to focus on where the plane needs to go and allow the flight control system to figure out how to control the plane so that it goes there. The solution lies in designing a control system that repeatedly "perturbs" the aircraft to analyze the current flight dynamics. As the plane flies along, the control system intentionally jiggles the aircraft again and again to see what happens. Sensors measure how the aircraft responds to each jiggle, and the control system uses that information to recalculate a model of the aircraft's response to its environment. The control system then uses that updated model when the pilot suddenly needs to execute a maneuver. Experienced healthcare providers essentially do the same thing when they titrate medications to manage a patient in the intensive care unit or in an operating room. They may not create a mathematical model, but they start to learn each patient's unique response. They use that information to modify the next dose.

Often, healthcare practitioners have to figure out if the patient's control system itself has stopped working properly. When a provider gets a hematocrit test on a patient, they are asking the laboratory to find out if the patient has the normal or expected percentage of their blood made up by red blood cells. If the percentage falls below what we consider normal, we would say the patient has anemia. The patient's body has a physiological control system that tries to keep the volume of red cells in that normal range, but something has gone wrong. Healthcare practitioners have learned a list of possible reasons for the body to have such a failure. To correct the problem, we need to know what went wrong, and that means we need to make a diagnosis. But what is the best way to proceed?

Strategy A might consist of testing for the most dangerous potential diagnosis first. Strategy B might consist of doing first a test for the most common cause of anemia. Strategy C might call for doing the least expensive test that would eliminate the highest number of potential causes. Strategy D might have the practitioner first do the test that has the highest reimbursement from the patient's medical insurance. Strategy E would have the practitioner first do the test that would immediately confirm the practitioner's guess for the correct diagnosis. In my experience Strategy E has a high number of subscribers. I would love to provide the reader with insight into the right answer to this question. I cannot. I tend to like Strategy C, but I also like Strategy A. Perhaps the real insight would be, "Medical practice can easily become tricky."

Chapter 8 Time Out

Perspicacity delves deeply beyond just the facts.
Does it perhaps separate the docs from the quacks?
You will need to make your own decision,
'Cause this book only lays out the basic collision.

We will explore **perspicacity** with examples in several more chapters of this book. Still, you might benefit from a quick step back at this point. You learned that Jonas Salk exhibited this trait of **perspicacity** when he suggested that focusing on the causes of cancer ultimately would not help mankind. Instead, he argued that we should research why everyone did not have this disease. It has taken medical science many decades to finally do what Salk recommended long ago.

Individuals involved in medical science include a great many scientists who stay away from the direct clinical care of patients. These folks get lumped into a medical science category that we commonly call the "basic sciences." Histologists, anatomists, physiologists, organic chemists, pharmacologists, and molecular biologists all fall into this group. It would seem fair to say these people rely more upon deductive reasoning in their work than the inductive tradition of medical therapy.

My medical career bounced about to include academic practice, private practice, and medical device manufacturing. My last job before I retired took me back to the academic realm, taking care of patients with resident physicians who were developing their clinical skills. In that educational institution, I was invited to join the Intellectual

Property Committee because of my previous experience working in the medical device industry.

The Committee met each month to make recommendations to the Dean on the wisdom of investments in inventions created by the various members of the staff. The medical school had ownership of the intellectual property arising from the efforts of its scientific staff. The Dean wanted to promote creativity and to share the rewards so that everyone would have a robust incentive to hatch ideas.

In the medical device industry, people from hospitals and medical schools brought their ideas to us, hoping to see their inventions become widely distributed products. The medical school wanted me on their Committee to help them understand how manufacturers might evaluate their ideas. I loved serving on this Committee. I looked forward each month to the afternoon that I would spend listening to astute members of the staff present their notions. Often, I heard ideas that I could not understand because they arose from details of medical knowledge I had never heard before. I was always fascinated.

Still, the thing that truly surprised me derived from the membership of the Intellectual Property Committee. Of the eight members, I alone had an M.D. degree. Every other member represented one of the basic science disciplines within the medical school. M.D. degree holders greatly outnumbered the Ph.D. holders within the institution. Clinicians brought ideas to the Committee, but clinicians were less willing to serve on the Committee. Indeed, the clinicians who brought ideas to the Committee often felt they received harsh treatment. The basic scientists perceived the clinicians' proposals as lacking the rigor needed to demonstrate their value. In truth, the clinicians mostly came with schemes for solving a problem instead of bringing proven solutions. Clinicians lacked the resources to develop and test their theories. The basic scientists literally spent all of their energy developing and validating new ideas. These differing perspectives lead to persistent friction that I could understand but rarely dispel.

This tale of the Intellectual Property Committee holds significance in our appreciation of **perspicacity**. Remember the definition of **perspicacity** as having a deep insight into a subject, akin to shrewdness. **Perspicacity** perhaps has greater importance in the basic sciences of medicine than in the delivery of patient care, since doing the right thing far outweighs knowing the reason. But in this book, we contend that searching more deeply for the "why" ultimately does impact delivering the best patient care.

Dr. Hill read my draft of this section of the book and reminded me that Medical Investigation 101 contains a paragraph paying tribute to Sakichi Toyoda. Toyoda, a renowned Japanese inventor, and industrialist founded Toyota. He wrote, "There is nothing that can't be done. If you can't make something, it's because you haven't tried hard enough." Toyoda believed that to find creative solutions, one must dig down to the root of the problem. To do that, he recommended a trick of thinking called "**5 Whys.**" Ask why, and then subject the answer to another level of asking why. Continue that process five times if you can. You can experiment with this exercise in the **perspicacity** examples that follow.

Chapter 9 How Does the Body Know It Has Been Injured?

Pain seems to protect the human body,
When hurt we stay home from Karate.
We need to give injuries time to heal,
But what exactly do we feel in this ordeal?

The resident physicians I helped train during my career were learning to practice the specialty of anesthesiology. Many consider the discovery of general anesthesia to represent America's most significant contribution to medical science. Surgeons treated patients for centuries before anyone discovered how to render people insensitive to pain. Today we can barely imagine how gruesome surgery must have played out then. We do know that operations then always took place in buildings distant from any other patients. No one wanted to hear the evidence of such agony. Let's not dwell on that image.

The first well documented general anesthetic was administered by William T. G. Morton on October 16, 1846, in Boston, Massachusetts. Historians have suggested that Morton had an unsavory reputation. We might not have expected that of a man who made such a significant advance in medical science. Nevertheless, mankind greatly appreciates the era of sophisticated surgical treatment advances that he initiated. Indeed, his gift still keeps on giving.

Anesthesiologists consider themselves consultants in perioperative medicine and experts in the relief of pain. One would, therefore, expect anesthesia residents to effortlessly answer the question that serves as the title of this chapter. Often when I worked with a new resident in the operating room, I would ask her or him that very question.

Their answer would usually start very much like this. "Injury or inflammation stimulates pain receptors on nerve endings." Next, they would invariably incorporate a mention of Substance P in their answer. Substance P has been a topic of intense medical research. My residents wanted to make sure I understood they were keeping up with the literature. I also have read numerous articles about Substance P, but I still do not understand the role it plays. Einstein said, "If you can't explain it to a six-year-old, you don't understand it yourself." I cannot explain Substance P to anyone.

The original question I asked them seems elementary. Indeed, my residents probably should have asked me how the patient's nerves knew the surgeon incised their skin. How can a nerve ending figure out that some tissue near it has been injured? [A nerve ending consists of a receptor, a structure, at the far end of a nerve that initiates signals in that nerve.] Clearly, specific nerves send messages to the brain that let us know very quickly if a surgeon or an enemy with a knife cuts our skin. But how does the nerve recognize that event?

My residents would ponder my question. Some decided that the knife must also cut the nerve, and that event triggered the sensation of pain. I stopped them as soon as they started that line of thinking. Each of them knew precisely the consequence of cutting a nerve. Cutting a nerve creates numbness. In some cases, a severed nerve can regenerate, and in other instances, that numbness becomes permanent. Cutting a nerve definitely does not produce pain.

At this point, I would suggest that we evaluate our options. Does the nerve detect injury chemically or physically? Physically seems unlikely because the pain persists long after the physical aspects of the insult go away. A chemical messenger seems more likely. Now we are exhibiting some **perspicacity**!

If a specific chemical acts as the messenger of tissue injury, the injury must bring that chemical in contact with the nerve ending. A receptor on the end of the nerve fiber would then recognize the damage. The receptor must excite the nerve when the messenger chemical contacts it. Now we only need to figure out the name of the messenger chemical.

It might help to figure out other requirements for this messenger molecule:

• We sense injuries very quickly and very reliably, so the messenger must exist in quantity all the time in every cell.

• The damage can release but not create the messenger for us to meet our criteria of speed and reliability.

• The messenger cannot exist outside of cells because then we would have pain continuously.

• A means might exist to rid this substance outside of cells within a few days. Our wounds stop hurting in that time frame.

It turns out that Dr. Geoffrey Burnstock, a British neurobiologist, figured all of this out in the early 1970s. However, other scientists questioned his findings for quite a few years. Burnstock identified adenosine triphosphate (ATP) as the messenger of tissue injury. ATP provides the energy to power all activities inside living cells. A specific enzyme present in the fluid outside of cells will destroy ATP, as we expected. ATP exists in large quantities inside of cells, so if a cell ruptures, the nerve ending has no trouble getting the message.

The story becomes even more fascinating as we dig deeper. Receptors to ATP, like those on the end of pain-sensing nerves, also exist on the surface of platelets. Coming in contact with ATP notifies platelets to get busy and create a clot to stop bleeding. We recognize that cells in human tissue grow in sheets, with each cell touching similar cells that surround it. It would seem logical to suppose that if we tugged on the structure excessively, cells would pull apart along their membranes. But if that were the case, a sprained ankle would not hurt because cells would not release ATP.

In truth, cells have tiny filament structures that pass through the membranes that cover them and reach deeply into the substance of their neighbors on all sides. Indeed, the binding of cells to each other has more complexity than I have suggested. One can spend many hours studying what anatomists know about cell-cell adhesion. In summary, if you tug hard enough on a tissue to pull cells apart, they actually rupture rather than separate with their covering membrane intact. A sprain does hurt!

I did not learn in medical school that cells will come apart (rupture) before they separate from each other. I did learn two facts that should have led me to that conclusion, but I ignored them. I learned that cancer metastasizes. And I learned that if you suck cells up into a syringe with a needle (called a fine needle biopsy), any unruptured ones are cancerous. When pathologists examine fine needle aspirates, healthy cells have all burst into fragments. Cancerous cells lack those tubular structures found in the healthy cells. Therefore, cancer cells can break off and wander to other places in the body, a behavior called metastasis.

Patients who have suffered trauma or surgery commonly find that becoming mobile and flexible again requires effort. As they heal, they experience considerable recurring discomfort over days, if not weeks. Why does this happen?

Let's try imagining ourselves as a cell inside the injured tissue. We recognize that we no longer have healthy cells surrounding us, so we know to initiate cell divisions to fill those voids. But we probably do not know precisely in what directions we need to aim our healing efforts.

Therefore, our healing process may send new cells into incorrect spots. Bending and twisting pull at those cells that have healed into the wrong locations. Pulling ruptures cells, releases ATP, and leads to pain. So, we have created a visual process model that could explain why healing has episodes of discomfort as we try to restore normal movement following trauma. We have exercised **perspicacity** in creating this explanation.

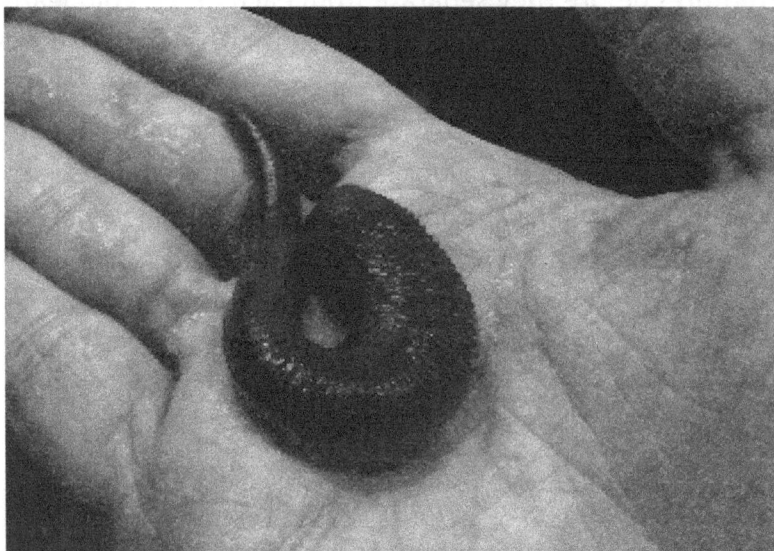

In 1951, Humphrey Bogart and Katharine Hepburn made a movie entitled "The African Queen." In that film, Bogart comes out of the water covered with leeches after pulling a boat through a swamp. Leeches can bite a significant hole in a person's skin (to suck out blood) without the victim feeling the injury. How do they do that? Would you believe the leech has an enzyme in its saliva that destroys ATP while it slowly nibbles its way through Humphrey Bogart's skin? Biologists actually discovered that enzyme in leech saliva well before Burnstock figured out its real function. The biologists had guessed the enzyme was present in the leech to keep platelets from clotting during the sucking of blood. (I apologize for the disgusting image.) They also knew that leech saliva contains an anticoagulant called Hirudin, but still did not guess the real function of the enzyme that deactivated ATP.

Acting with **perspicacity**, we might wonder if surgeons could use enzymes that destroy ATP (such enzymes we call ATPases) to make surgery painless. I like that idea a lot, although apparently, surgeons would need to operate very, very slowly. Leeches must bite their victims gradually to allow the enzyme time to remove all the ATP. Most surgeons do not have the patience of a leech. If surgeons washed out their incisions with an ATPase before closing wounds, might patients recover without pain? That approach might have merit, but the ATP may also play a role both in blood clotting and in wound healing. So, we need more research to feed our **perspicacity**.

I hope you are impressed by how this **perspicacity** has led to a variety of intriguing possibilities. That would not have come about if we had not asked how our nervous system recognizes tissue injury.

Let's allow our **perspicacity** to take us one more step. If a Leech has an ATPase in its saliva that keeps its victim comfortable while being bitten, might humans also have something similar in our saliva? Wound licking behavior exists. Over the ages human have found some benefit in "licking their wounds." Researchers have found factors in saliva that may promote healing and other agents that play an antibacterial role. I found a paper that reports human saliva contains more than 3,000 different proteins, but I could not find clear evidence that we have in that mix an effective enzyme that would destroy ATP in a wound. But would the caveman have "licked his wounds" to fight off infection? No. But to reduce the pain? Absolutely.

The word "shrewdness" appears in the definition of **perspicacity**. Let's focus on that for a moment. We say someone displays shrewdness when they see a dimension of a situation that others may not appreciate. When I asked resident physicians about how the body detects an injury, they would quickly recognize that they really did not know. I would ask them if that was ever discussed in their medical school lectures. They said no. They had never seen that addressed in their textbooks either. I would then ask if they would conclude that no one knew how this happens. They would usually agree with that conclusion.

If we were to search the medical literature diligently and not find the answer to a question like this one, can we conclude that no one knows the answer? It turns out that you can actually watch Burnstock talk about ATP as the messenger of tissue injury on YouTube. Burnstock does not talk about whether or not an enzyme that destroys ATP would interfere with wound healing. I have not found the answer to that question in the medical literature. Does that mean that no one knows the answer to that question? Can I get you to say yes?

How would a shrewd medical scientist answer that question? He or she would say, "There are people who know the answers to questions like this one but are contractually blocked from telling us what they know." What? Who are they? Why do they not publish their discovery? Science should not work that way.

The answer lies in the domain of intellectual property. If a company, institute, or university hopes to market a medication or a methodology of treatment, they invest money in research to answer such questions. They hire scientists to figure out how to solve a particular problem. They ask these researchers to sign a contract saying they will keep their knowledge secret until they have defined their concept enough to file patents on their insights and methods. Healthcare practitioners commonly have little awareness of this community of medical scientists who know these secrets.

I was fortunate to work at one time in my career with a very shrewd clinical researcher. When he got interested in a new medical research topic he would get on an airplane and go visit other researchers in that field. Before he even planned his own research, he would discuss it with colleagues. He would have read publications written by those colleagues, but he argued that was not enough. He said, "No one publishes the experiments they did that failed, but they will tell you about them if you go and ask. I don't want to reproduce what they did that gave them new insights. I also do not want to pursue ideas they already know do not answer the crucial questions. You can only learn about the failed experiments that wasted their time if you show up at their laboratory." Perspicacious medical scientists put that lesson into their bag of tricks.

Chapter 10 Medical Misadventures

The fact that therapy can go very wrong,
Deserves no poem, just a sad, sad song.
Folks electing careers in patient care,
Do it to make life a lot more fair.

The path to a career in medical science requires a considerable amount of grit. No one makes the grade effortlessly. No one travels through without setbacks and self-doubts. So why put oneself through that torture. Some may start down that road looking for respect, a rewarding profession, the challenge of unraveling mysteries, or simply a chance to help others. A part of everyone's motivation may stem from a basic appreciation that illness and injury seem to happen randomly, and medical care seeks to restore fairness. Certainly, some people appear to bring poor health upon themselves through neglect or bad decisions. But even then, we see others live similar lives without misfortune. If we think everyone has a right to healthcare, we believe that because healthcare seems to take us closer to justice for all.

If a blunder in the delivery of healthcare results in a bad outcome from one's medical therapy, that event seems to layer one injustice atop another. We might call that "double jeopardy," the very opposite of justice. And yet it happens.

No one can accurately count the mistakes made in the delivery of healthcare. We do not expect the treatment of patients to always prove successful. But researchers can document errors, and they have published papers suggesting that more than 30,000 people die in American hospitals each year as a consequence of errors. The exact number might exceed ten times that figure, depending upon which investigator does the counting. I considered pulling together a summary of the various published studies, but instead decided to focus on errors from the care provider's perspective.

No one can make it through a career as a healthcare provider without making mistakes. Humans make mistakes. A few of those errors will injure patients. Both ill-conceived actions, or a failure to act can harm. During their training, students rely on their teachers to keep everyone safe as they learn to provide care to patients. Eventually, the day arrives for every student when no one else stands between a decision and its consequences, both good and bad. Each of us who decides to treat human patients must deal with that ominous burden. But everyone who travels that path has allies.

I could write about my experiences of making decisions that did not go well. I might try to describe the agony of self-doubt those events engendered. Or, I could tell you about the amazing, experienced cardiac surgeon who, late one evening, dragged me away from a patient's intensive care bedside into a conference room. At the bedside, I had confessed doubt about a therapeutic choice I made during the earlier surgery. This surgeon, twice my age, proceeded in private to lecture me sternly. He said he was happy to talk to me about my decisions, but he would not allow me to suggest that we had not both done the very best we could have done for this struggling patient. I never forgot that lecture. That is what I mean about having allies when you take up this burden. I was at the beginning of my career, and I was feeling the stress of being alone to make irreversible decisions that affected the lives of human beings. But I was not alone on that journey.

I remember today every detail of several cases that did not go well years ago in my career. I wish I had made some decisions differently. I do not know if those different decisions would have changed the outcome. Nonetheless, I regret the decisions I made. Everyone who does these jobs lives with those experiences. The joy of actions we took that saved lives tends to make our choice to do this work worthwhile, but in quiet moments the good decisions never seem to totally crowd out the questionable ones.

I will tell you about an experience in my career that illustrates how people with the best of intentions can make a mistake that haunts them later. But after that, I want to talk about a future where mistakes will shrink away.

Patients often need to have their gallbladders removed because lumps form inside and block the passage of liver bile into the intestine. The reason for this condition still remains mysterious, but treatment necessitates surgery. Years ago, the surgery required a significant incision made just below the lowest rib on the right side of the abdomen. Now surgeons can remove the gallbladder through tiny incisions using a laparoscope. Before the arrival of the laparoscope, recovery from gallbladder surgery involved considerable discomfort. Every deep breath pulled at injured muscles along that lower rib. A physician colleague and I read back then about a method to make local anesthesia last for more than a day, instead of just hours. That duration could allow us to make the recovery from gallbladder surgery much more comfortable. We showed the hospital pharmacist the published recipe for this concoction. He agreed to mix a specific local anesthetic with medicinal dextran so we could deaden the nerves to this area for many hours to benefit our patients.

We used this mixture perhaps a dozen times and grew very excited by the results. About this time, a general surgeon called me late in the afternoon to say he needed to do urgent gallbladder surgery for a patient who had come into the emergency room during the day. I visited the woman to evaluate her for surgery. This 52-year-old woman seemed very sick. Normally she enjoyed good health and lived an active lifestyle. I told her I planned to administer a general anesthetic and that I would block the nerves between her ribs with our "magic" mixture to keep her comfortable following the procedure.

The surgical procedure went smoothly. The patient's stay in the recovery room seemed routine. The next afternoon, I went her hospital room to see her. I expected to find her resting comfortably because of our miracle nerve block. Instead, she felt miserable, feeling constant pain. She could not rest despite receiving repeated high doses of narcotics from the nurses. I examined her abdomen and found she seemed to have residual numbness of the skin around her bandage from the nerve block. I was confused. Previous patients having our special nerve block had reported remarkable comfort.

I wrote a note on the patient's chart documenting my findings and the fact that I could not explain her degree of discomfort. The block still rendered her abdominal wall numb. I knew the surgeon would be seeing her soon, and I wanted to make him aware of my concern and my confusion.

The following day I learned that the patient had died during the night from a ruptured aortic aneurysm. The aorta, the body's largest artery, had ruptured so suddenly that no intervention could have spared her life.

How could such a thing happen? The patient came to the hospital with abdominal pain consistent with several possible causes. An ultrasound examination of her abdomen found gallstones that would explain her symptoms. That examination might have picked up an aortic aneurysm, but no one saw that. We acted on a proven diagnosis, but we missed the additional diagnosis that threatened and ultimately took her life. My nerve block was ineffective because her pain was coming from blood leaking from her aorta, not from the surgical wound. As a team, we failed this patient. We made a diagnosis that appeared to fit her symptoms, but we did not rule out every alternative diagnosis that we could and should have considered.

The mistakes that can occur during hospital care can fill a very long list. Patients can get medications at the wrong time, in the wrong dose, or even the wrong medication. Patients can fail to receive essential medications. They may have a test that fails to pick up an abnormality. The staff may fail to recognize the significance of a specific result. Communications can go astray. The patient can slip and fall in the hospital. The patient can get a new infection while inside the hospital. All of these things and many more fall into the category of medical errors. We label all infections that begin inside the hospital as mistakes, even if we find no specific mistake that lead to the infection. Deciding if a mistake contributed to harm often requires someone to make a judgment that different experts might dispute. For that reason, researchers differ on what counts as a mistake. Everyone does agree that mistakes occur.

This topic belongs in a book about **perspicacity** in medical science because, as we approach the end of three decades of attention to this problem, conventional thinking has not solved it. We need a shrewd new perspective. Let's review what hospitals have attempted to do to reduce mistakes.

Even before medical mistakes became a topic of wide public concern in 1990, each hospital medical specialty conducted monthly Morbidity and Mortality Conferences. In these meetings, the professional staff reviewed all major complications that patients experienced during their care.

Often these meetings prompted quite a lively debate among practitioners. Colleagues readily disagreed with decisions as they searched for the best treatments. The intent lay in finding work processes that would prevent future recurrence of specific complications. Commonly this objective proved elusive.

Originally records were kept of the Morbidity and Mortality Conference discussions so that hospital inspectors could see that the medical staff was doing everything possible to reduce untoward events. *[Morbidity means the condition of being diseased and mortality means the condition of being dead.]* At some point, lawyers discovered that they could get copies of these discussions from state health departments to use in lawsuits on behalf of injured patients. Hospitals quickly stopped keeping records of these meetings. Some changed the name of the meetings to something more akin to a "Quality Conference" instead of the more evocative title "Morbidity and Mortality." They wanted to make clear that their future discussions were educational and should remain private to best benefit society.

Hospitals created separate internal teams to conduct formal root cause analysis investigations of their mishaps. These teams would take responsibility for decreasing mistakes by developing fault-tolerant work processes. State and federal governments used inspections and a variety of management tools to reduce mistakes in healthcare. Organizations have created extensive training for quality improvement in healthcare. The Federal Government has promoted publicly reported ratings of hospital performance to create a strong incentive for error reduction. Many hospitals have implemented management initiatives dubbed "A Culture of Safety." These efforts have been earnest, intensive, well supported, and effective in making many changes that have benefited society. But no one would argue that the problem has gone away.

Some have argued that medical science can never achieve the quality measures that manufacturers like Motorola have famously achieved. Medical experts reason that each patient differs from every other one, while manufacturers make the identical product over and over again. This difference, they argue, means we cannot simply apply the same strategy used in manufacturing to the hospital.

Bear in mind, the therapy for almost every medical condition improves over time. Some have argued that medical mishaps become more dangerous because the therapy has become more potent. For example, if we had no good treatment for a specific condition, we could not judge anything we tried as an error. When we have highly effective therapies, we perceive failure of the treatment as a mistake. Similarly, it seems more difficult to avoid medication errors when we have 10,000 different medications. When we had less than 500 prescription medications, we had fewer opportunities for mistakes.

The effort to reduce mistakes has hatched several oft-repeated axioms. The axioms themselves appear to contain flaws:

• You cannot fix what you cannot measure. (Of course, you can. You can fix a leaky faucet without measuring the quantity of the leak.)

• Only healthcare professionals can fix this problem because only they understand the details of patient care. (We will soon consider some approaches to error reduction that healthcare professionals do not have the expertise to use effectively.)

• Since physicians best understand the appropriate treatments, healthcare works best when physicians write orders that others carry out precisely. (We will present evidence to challenge this traditional mode of medical practice.)

• The only way to deal with the expanding complexity of medical science lies in making smaller and smaller areas of expertise, so-called sub-sub-specialists. (Eventually we might have physicians who only treat patients with a lesion of the right eyebrow. This approach would appear to make medicine more similar to the Motorola environment, but it has not played out so successfully. If a patient mistakenly gets a referral to the wrong sub-sub-specialist, serious problems can readily ensue.)

Should we give up all hope? Has anyone applied **perspicacity** to move this effort in a novel, positive (safer) direction? Yes, they have. Indeed, I persist in believing that the next generation of medical scientists will make great strides in the elimination of errors in medical care despite our meager improvements over the last three decades. Let's examine this possibility.

I would nominate Dr. Lawrence Weed, M.D. (1923 - 2017), as the poster image of **perspicacity** within the ranks of practicing physicians. Larry Weed, by his own admission, was never popular with his colleagues. As a Professor of Internal Medicine at the University of Vermont, he frequently irritated his associates with his dissatisfaction with the status quo. Recognizing that physicians might easily forget one or two problems amongst many issues in a patient's condition, Weed created the "Problem Oriented Patient Record." He disrupted the traditional organization of the medical chart. The acceptance of this new format emerged slowly, but today it has become a mandated standard in American hospitals.

Weed's system requires that the chart contain a list of all the patient's medical problems. Each problem gets a date or origination and a date of resolution. Without a resolution date the problem remains active. All progress notes in the chart must reference a specific problem by its number on the list. The patient's physicians should never again overlook a problem because it will remain active on the list until definitively resolved.

Dr. Weed also lectured audiences on a separate cause of mistakes that he observed in medical care. While medical students were taught to conduct patient interviews and examinations in a very systematic, thorough fashion, he found that his residents took shortcuts. He hated seeing this happen. Instead of going through a thorough array of questions and examination steps, his residents would guess a diagnosis after hearing the patient barely begin to relate their complaints. Once the resident had guessed a presumed diagnosis, he or she would only ask questions or investigate signs that would confirm their presumption. While the resident saw this strategy as a boon to efficiency, Weed saw it as a grand opportunity for error and harm to the patient, not unlike the mistaken gallbladder surgery I discussed earlier in this chapter.

Dr. Weed conducted a fascinating experiment to verify his observation. He recruited several nurses to take histories and do a preliminary examination of the patients on his service before they were seen by his resident physicians. The nurses were only asked to create a problem list, and not to make any diagnosis. He taught them the thorough, classical method of taking a complete history. He also taught them how to conduct a thorough basic physical examination. He then compared the problem lists written by his nurses with those written by his residents. He reported in one of his recorded lectures that the nurses listed four times as many problems as did his residents. Furthermore, he reported that his residents listed items on their problem lists that were not valid problems. For example, one resident wrote on the list, "Rule out MI." The patient did not complain to the physician that he wanted to make sure he was not having a heart attack. The patient probably complained of chest discomfort. The resident decided to make sure the patient was not having a myocardial infarction (MI). That intent appears praiseworthy, but if one defines the problem that way, finding no MI would cancel the problem and stop any further search for a cause of the patient's pain. Apparently, the resident also collected no further information from the patient to help find the true source of the pain. In essence, the resident had "put all his eggs in one little basket."

Apparently jumping to a conclusion does not only occur with resident physicians in their training. Numerous studies suggest that practicing physicians commonly decide on a diagnosis within seconds of starting to listen to the patient's complaint. But we have not found all the causes of mistakes. Dr. Peter Pronovost, while an Anesthesiologist and Intensive Care Specialist at Johns Hopkins, conducted a very different experiment to reduce errors. (Dr. Pronovost earned international notoriety for eliminating dangerous central line infections, but we are going to focus here on yet another insightful concept he pursued.)

Typically, physicians make rounds on their patients and then write orders for the nursing staff and various technicians to carry out to treat their patients. I am going to call that method of practice "prescriptive." Dr. Pronovost decided to modify this approach in his intensive care unit by requiring that physicians always make rounds with a senior nurse from the unit. As they made rounds, the nurse was told to create with the physician a statement of the objective of their therapy for each patient for that day. They had to agree on that statement before they moved on to see the next patient. The objective had to contain one or more demonstrable goals for each patient to achieve by the end of the day. The physicians still had to write their customary orders, but they also now had to set goals for the therapy.

For example, perhaps the physician wanted to get his patient being managed on a ventilator to be breathing on his own by the end of the day. That would constitute a clear therapy goal. The nurse would write that goal on a whiteboard at the head of the patient's bed so that everyone involved with the patient knew the goal. That does not seem like a significant change, but the results proved startling. The physicians immediately found they were getting telephone calls in high numbers. A nurse might phone to say that it appeared the pain medications ordered for the patient were in conflict with the goal and ask for that order to be modified. The physical therapist might call to ask permission to modify their passive motion treatments to a different set to assist getting the patient off the ventilator. You get the idea. Everyone started using their skills to get the patient to the objective, instead of simply carrying out the physician's written orders. Pronovost showed this process produced faster recovery and fewer complications. Apparently collaborative goal setting outperforms conventional prescriptive care.

Dr. Brent James at Intermountain Healthcare in Utah also has used **perspicacity** to advance safer, more effective hospital care. Dr. James recognized early in his career as a surgeon that finding the best therapy for any specific medical problem seemed impossible. The medical literature supported a variety of options. Polling six experts commonly resulted in six or more suggestions. Within an institution, treatments varied so widely no one could reliably evaluate the outcomes for any specific approach. After exhaustive study, Dr. James proposed a plan that won the support of the health maintenance organization where he worked. They picked several common medical conditions and formed small teams to write protocols for care in those situations guided by the best information they could find. They did not require members of the medical staff to use the protocols. Instead, they insisted that physicians modify the protocol to fit the needs of their patient, or write a quick note letting the team know why the protocol did not meet their patient's needs. The team was required to meet every six months to update the protocol based on the modifications physicians were making or based on medical advances. Dr. James told everyone from the beginning that at the very best a protocol could only meet the needs of 85% of patients without modifications. They would always expect their medical staff to adjust every protocol to the unique circumstances of the patient.

Each year Intermountain Health added more protocols and modified previous ones. Physicians who elected at first to never use protocols quietly changed their practice as colleagues began to achieve better results using them. The fact that the protocols lead to more consistent care allowed the institution to see more opportunities for improvement. Intermountain Health began to find that the protocols reduced complications and brought down costs. Better outcomes cost less! Working from a protocol while adapting it for unique situations meant less opportunity for errors of omission in therapy.

Dr. Brent James did not originate his highly effective strategy sitting by himself in an empty room. No. He started out earning a degree in electrical engineering. After becoming a surgeon, he earned a master's degree in statistics to further his quest for the path to higher quality in medical care. Other fields of science have contributed significantly to the quest for quality and error reduction. Dr. Donald Norman came at this issue by studying psychology. His book, "The Design of Everyday Things," opened a door in the design community that plays a crucial role in error reduction. Norman coined the concept of "putting information into the world" as a substitute for reliance on training or memory to improve performance. The protocols Brent James created at Intermountain Healthcare represent an example of putting information into the world. Instead of having physicians start the care of each patient with a blank sheet of paper, the protocol provides a template for creating a unique plan for a unique patient. In other words, it puts information into the world that the physician then adjusts.

In the industrial design sphere, putting information into the world means that products and processes should suggest, or even force the user to perform without mistakes because of the design. The design has built into it the information needed for correct utilization. The best design for a product, a tool, or a process should need no instruction manual because the design should make proper use visible to the user.

Donald Norman played a leadership role in Apple Computer's Advanced Technology Group. There he relentlessly fought for the notion that the designer should build the solutions to problems into the product so that the customer could focus entirely on their objective. That philosophy had a great deal to do with the success of the Apple Computer. Customers quickly discovered they could use these computers without a degree in computer science. In this same manner the design community has a great deal to offer medical science in the quest to reduce mistakes. They do this today by virtue of being involved in the design of medical devices. Ideally these skills should move into the design of the process of medical practice itself. This has started. Industrial Designs at GE Healthcare have designed the "experience" for children needing a Magnetic Resonance Imaging examination so that they do not need sedation to comfortably hold still for a scan. That accomplishment represents only the beginning of what we might see from the design community.

Sean Hagen heads a design firm that works primarily in the medical device arena. Sean himself has written and lectured extensively on the topic of "conceptual observation." Industrial designers long ago recognized that one could not understand the subtle features of a process or task simply by asking questions. Individuals who perform a task do not always recognize the precise sequence of their actions. Often, they may do a key step without awareness. Even when they have expertise, they may not appreciate all the integrated details when it comes to finding a better path to accomplishment. The designer may need to catalogue and dissect each tiny twist and turn of a task in order to meet a design objective.

The organized approach for doing this design work they call "conceptual observation," much of which they derived from the principles of ethnography in the field of anthropology. What does this look like? Industrial designers do a great deal of their work graphically: watching, taking photographs, making drawings, measuring, color coding diagrams of movement, looking from the inside out, turning the process upside down, etc. Hagen says that commonly when they present one of their investigations to medical clients, the healthcare professionals say they have never looked at their procedures in such detail. They then ask if they should be viewing all their techniques with such intensity. Probably so, in the name of **perspicacity**. More reasonably, medical providers could form continuing partnerships with industrial designers because this type of analysis requires a specific set of practiced skills.

I would like to add one more comment about the work of Dr. Brent James and the power of his protocol system. The protocols clearly augment the memory of the physicians for up-to-date details of treatment options, especially useful for rare conditions. Intermountain Health implements the protocols on their hospital information system's computers. Computer implementation would allow protocols to include computational algorithms to further guide therapy. Researchers have shown that such algorithms can use multiple pieces of patient information to arrive at dosing recommendations that dramatically decrease complications from therapy. Algorithms have been proven highly effective in dosing pain medications, but potentially have more extensive uses. Clinicians may not have the time and energy to work through complex decision trees to find the optimal dosing, but computers do not seem to object. In the coming years we should expect much more frequent use of computers and learning algorithms to contribute to the safety and sophistication of our healthcare system.

Chapter 11 Physical Examination

The detail complaints of a patient are told,
So, the doc can make a diagnosis unfold.
The doc can add physical examination clues,
But hopefully it all spells "no bad news."

We started this book with the notion that the fire hydrant flow of information in medical education squeezes out any time for serious reflection and creativity, not to mention a social life. Practitioners in patient care face an overwhelming amount of work required to get them into a high state of proficiency for treating patients. Memorizing essential knowledge erases much musing over the "whys" and "how comes." No wonder most big breakthroughs in medical science arise from the efforts of basic scientists rather than medical practitioners. That result may not imply a problem, but it could suggest a missed opportunity for process improvement in health care delivery. To that end, in this chapter we will take a quick look at the process of physical examination of patients in a doctor's office.

As second year medical students we were paired with a fellow student for practical instruction in physical examination. My partner had been a very successful football linebacker in his college years. Therefore, my first experiences using a stethoscope and percussing an abdomen reminded me of a time that I painted a barn. My cooperative partner wore at least size XXXL and his muscle mass, as I recall, matched the rigidity and size of that barn.

The examination seemed more like geological study than biological. I listened to his heart sounds and breath sounds as instructed in the exercise. He did the same on my smaller, less imposing physique. I did a great deal of stethoscope listening for decades thereafter, probably adding up to thousands of hours. I admit I never felt like I ranked as accomplished in that skill. I never felt absolutely sure I heard a heart murmur unless it rattled windows and doors.

What are we really doing in this ritual of the physical examination? I was taught originally that we were gathering evidence to guide us to a correct diagnosis of a patient's illness or injury. As an anesthesiologist, I more often had to diagnose the effects of drugs I had given the patient myself, but I used a stethoscope constantly in doing that. I took blood pressures and I examined patients routinely to evaluate their status and their response to my treatments. But I was not using the physical examination the same way an internist would apply his or her more practiced skills.

I wear glasses. I have visited an optometrist or ophthalmologist annually for decades. When I first got glasses as a child, the ophthalmologist put individual lenses in front of my eyes sequentially asking me if that lens made my vision better or worse. That process seemed to go on a long time. Now when I visit the ophthalmologist, his crew of technicians uses a half dozen high-tech instruments to measure and scan my eyes so that when the doctor finally pops into the process, he has screens and screens of information to review. That takes him about a minute. Then he checks out my retina using his slit lamp. I suspect that he does that slit lamp thing just to appear interested. Then we talk about the cows that he raises for a few minutes before I am sent home. He does not own a single stethoscope.

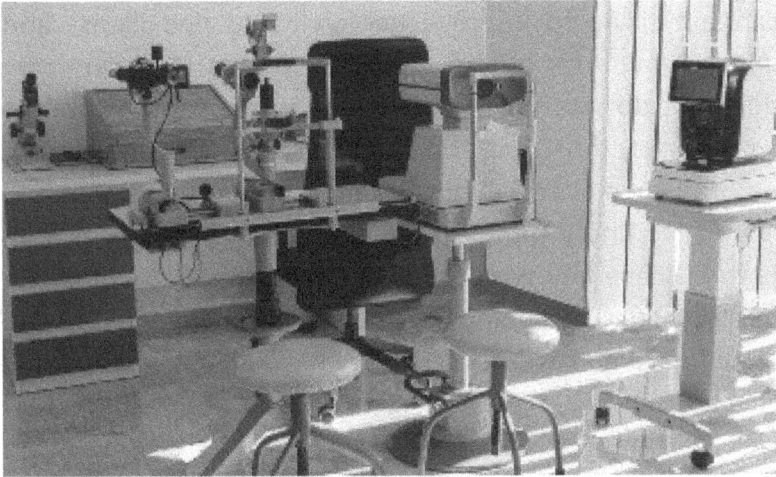

I also go to see my primary care physician at least annually. Her nurse puts me on a scale with all of my clothing and shoes still on. Then the nurse takes my blood pressure. My doctor talks to me at some length, primarily asking me to report on any symptoms I might have. She uses her stethoscope on my heart, lungs, and carotids. She pushes on my stomach and orders some blood tests. Then she tells me to exercise more. I wonder why she does not need as much equipment to check my entire body as my eye doctor requires to evaluate two small eyeballs.

I think my primary care physician received excellent training and does her job with competence. I believe she can and does use the physical examination to guide her diagnostic skills, but fortunately, I have not needed her to sort out any serious issues. Can I ask for anything more? Yes.

If I evoke some **perspicacity**, I would like to ask my primary care physician to improve her ability to find illness and injury in my body before I have symptoms. She currently does not do that well. She listens to my carotid arteries with her stethoscope and might detect some narrowing before I have a stroke, but her method has flaws. I would like her to find a tumor in my lung, liver, or pancreas long before I have any symptoms, but she cannot. I would like her to make sure I do not have an aortic aneurysm, but she would have no clue, especially if I have an aneurysm in my chest.

Perhaps you are thinking, "He wants too much." But should not the goal of primary care lie in detecting illness before it progresses to symptoms? Is it possible to do that?

Recently I read that the University of Connecticut Medical School is teaching all medical students how to use and interpret ultrasound imaging. Exciting! I believe that means that these medical students will go into practice knowing how to image my spleen and pancreas in their office and measure the wall thickness of my carotid arteries a few seconds later. Then they will check out my aorta from top to bottom. They will likely find conditions in my body that need attention before I report symptoms. They will generate images and measurements of my anatomy and physiology very much the way my eye doctor currently does for my eyes. They may even toss out their stethoscopes.

Other technologies may also come along in the future to increase our ability to predict pathology early enough to stop its progress. Ultrasound imaging should have come into wider use much sooner. It started as a tool for radiologists to use as an alternative to the X-ray. Obstetricians started to use this technology to examine the unborn fetus safely, and radiologists supported the migration of these machines into that specialty. Next, anesthesiologists began using ultrasound to locate nerves accurately to make regional anesthesia more reliable. At about the same time, they began using ultrasound probes placed into the esophagus during general anesthesia to watch the heart continuously during cardiac surgery. Recently, anesthesiologists have begun taking an ultrasound machine with them to cardiac emergencies within the hospital so that they can immediately see what the heart is doing. Soon we will have data on the success of this new use ultrasound, but early reports suggest it offers significant advantages in making resuscitation more effective.

Chapter 12 What is a virus?

If a cell were blown up to the size of a house,
A virus would seem 'bout the size of a mouse.
The cell has the means to live a full life,
But a virus has nothing but a tight coat and strife.

A great deal of the writing of this book took place during the COVID-19 Pandemic. People are sick around the world and dying from an illness caused by a virus. Where does a virus come from? A living organism hatched it, but why? Does it serve some useful purpose? We commonly do not expect any benefit to arise from any virus, ever. **Perspicacity** requires that we try somehow to imagine what it is like to be that virus.

That sounds like a very dismal assignment at best. If I am now a virus, how did I come about? What need did I fulfill? Killing innocent people around the world does not seem like a mission to take pride in accomplishing. How does evolution favor my arrival on this planet?

In the year 2020, probably more news stories have been written about the COVID-19 virus than any other subject. I have not seen a single item in the news suggesting any good has come about from this virus. So why does it exist? Perhaps a cosmic ray intersected with a benign, useful virus and changed it into COVID-19. Does a harmless, helpful virus ever occur?

Did COVID-19 happen by accident? This virus readily spreads from human to human. It invades human cells. It tricks those cells to reproduce more of the virus, and, in return, it then kills the cell. In that process, it also kills many people. Did it evolve for that specific role?

Who cares how it came about? We should care because understanding the 'why' might offer clues to help humans survive its attack. In a war, knowledge of the enemy always seems to aid the defenders.

A virus cannot reproduce itself, and as a consequence, biologists do not classify this protein sleeve with genetic material inside as "living." The story becomes enthralling when we look more deeply. A single teaspoon of seawater contains as many as 10,000,000 viruses. That seems impressive because we have quite a few teaspoons of seawater in our oceans. But consider this. Virologists estimate that each human being has over 100,000,000,000 viruses inside of us. One hundred trillion? That sounds ridiculous.

How does a massive number of viruses like that square with the common impression that viruses always cause disease? They must play a different role beyond causing illness and death. **Perspicacity** demands we dig deeper into what all of these viruses are doing inside healthy people.

Medical science does not have an established understanding of the origin of the virus. We have theories. Viruses may have come from complex molecules before living cells existed (the Virus First Hypothesis). They may have originated inside tiny one-cell organisms (the Reduction Hypothesis). Viruses may arise from snippets of genetic material that escape from the living cells of plants or animals (the Escape Hypothesis). None of these theories appear to mesh with all the facts. Observations that do not fit with our understanding of nature remind us of the problems that Albert Einstein found himself drawn to study in the realm of physics. Einstein sought a visual image to explain the riddles to better understand our universe. Ah! Perhaps we have in the virus a genuine challenge for the perspicacious medical scientist.

Jonas Salk would recommend that we imagine ourselves as a virus. We would want to establish an origin for ourselves as a virus. Did we have a parent? We were likely born via the talents and energy of a living cell, but what cell? A germ, a cell in a rose bush, or perhaps a cell in the trunk of an elephant? Once born, we do not need to grow or even propel ourselves to get about. We need no energy and thus have no need for food. We do contain a skill. We embody a length of DNA or RNA that codes for the manufacture of one or more chemical molecules that make progeny (copies of oneself) and may also make other substances. The perspective one achieves being a virus has intrigue. But we generated no immediate revelations.

If we search the literature on viruses, most of it will deal with the damage viruses do in this world. Thus, we have a difficult time liking ourselves while assuming the identity of a virus. But eventually, we might stumble upon a 2017 piece in the Annual Review of Virology entitled "The Good That Viruses Do." A glimmer of hope...

We could find a cheerleader singing the praises of reputable viruses in a 2020 book by Marilyn Roossinck entitled "Virus: An Illustrated Guide to 101 Incredible Microbes." Roossinck reports on viruses that appear to form cooperative relationships with plants and fungi. Her work suggests many more links of this sort may exist in the world, still not yet discovered. Others have suggested that the role of a virus might better be defined as a set of skills stored away in a steamer trunk for future use as needed. We know that we can find viruses that seem to be helpful to individual plants lounging about on the plant's surface. We find these viruses also inside the seeds of that plant. Could it be that we have mistakenly given the virus a bad rap when they really do a great deal of good?

Perhaps living organisms of all sorts shed snippets of their genetic material packaged up for survival in a protein or protein-lipid overcoat. The overcoat protects the DNA or RNA, but also gives the genetic coding the ability to return back into the nucleus of the cell type that spawned it. When all goes smoothly, the virus benefits the cell that spawned it. Perhaps a virus may get inside a cell accidentally that it never was intended to visit. Of course, it would try to pursue the task it was built to perform, although that activity may not work at all in the foreign host. In fact, this unexpected combination might turn out to look like the work of the devil. The next thing you know, the New York Times has printed headlines calling this tiny innocent virus trying to do its job a PANDEMIC! Mother nature seemingly can act lovingly at one moment and turn savage the next. The idea that deadly viruses may have a beneficial role elsewhere serves as a hypothesis for us to explore.

No one said a single kind word about germs or viruses in the infectious disease course in my medical school. I understand that the intent of that class lay in exposing the evil of disease, yet mankind might benefit from a different understanding of our partnership with the world of microbes. That understanding comes closer every year, and probably has benefits we cannot yet fully imagine.

The origin of the virus remains a mystery. Virologists spend their careers learning more and more about this entity. Yet despite knowing volumes about them, we still may have misunderstood the benefit they provide in nature. I encourage you to think further on this topic than I have been able to take you.

Chapter 13 What good is angina?

Angina means a crushing pain in the chest,
A pain that makes its victims distressed.
Usually, pain serves our self-interest as an alarm,
But angina actually tries to do us great harm.

Chest pain brings large numbers of patients to emergency rooms in America's hospitals. ERs have a carefully rehearsed choreography to manage this complaint quickly and efficiently because the problem can abruptly prove fatal. Before they diagnose the cause of the discomfort, they assume the patient is having a heart attack, technically referred to as a myocardial infarction. Those words mean that they suspect the patient's heart lacks enough oxygen somewhere in its muscle mass to keep up with the work of pumping blood throughout the patient's body. We know that inside the muscles of the heart, we have nerves that can detect inadequate levels of oxygen.   Health professionals refer to this oxygen deficit as ischemia.

Unfortunately, practitioners cannot count on chest pain to always signal a problem with the heart. Indeed, they cannot even rely on the patient feeling this ischemia in their chest. In some cases, they feel it in other parts of their body. Emergency room staff therefore treat lots of pains as cardiac until they make absolutely sure the patient does not have a problem with their heart. Since some patients feel ischemia in their heart as jaw pain, dentists often find heart attack patients coming into their office for treatment.

When the hospital staff suspects a heart attack, they want the patient to lie down to reduce the amount of work required to pump blood. They have the patient breathe pure oxygen, so the arterial blood carries more oxygen to the muscles. They give these patients an aspirin tablet to reduce the formation of clots inside of arteries that may be the cause of the problem. After those steps, they can proceed to figure out the actual problem using clues from EKGs, blood tests, and thorough medical histories.

Emergency room doctors also treat suspected heart attack patients with a dose of a strong narcotic, especially if they find the patient has an abnormally fast pulse rate and elevated blood pressure. Both a rapid pulse rate and a high blood pressure cause the heart to work harder, and that makes a heart attack more lethal. But the ischemia receptors in the heart cause a fast pulse rate and elevate the blood pressure when they sense trouble. In other words, ischemia receptors make the heart attack worse.

Emergency room staff need to use a narcotic to reverse the unwanted consequence of these receptors that we assume are there to benefit the patient. Why would human beings evolve nerve receptors that try to kill us when we have insufficient blood flow to our hearts? That seems wrong.

I learned about this problem in medical school, but no one asked our professor why. Instead, we took notes on the proper things to do for the patient. That included the use of a narcotic to protect the patient from his or her own nervous system. We failed at that moment to exercise **perspicacity**.

So, I am going to ask you. Why do we have receptors in our hearts that make the organ work harder at a time when they should lower the heart rate and lower the blood pressure to save our life? Perhaps you can put down this book for a few minutes and think about your answer. Perhaps a beverage might help your creative juices while you ponder this riddle. Take your time. Ask a friend.

You are back. You have pondered. Now you want to check the accuracy of your conclusion.

I must admit that I wrote down in my medical school notes that morphine could reduce the workload of the heart affected by cardiac ischemia. I did not immediately ask myself why this situation might arise. Several years later, a neurophysiologist told me that graduate students working in his lab had a running argument about this feature of human physiology. They initially decided that heart attacks usually happened after adults were past the age of having children. Perhaps evolution might prefer that heart attacks prove fatal at that age to reduce the total food needs of the tribe. This would help the younger members of the tribe have more children and create an evolutionary advantage. I had to agree this argument made sense, but it also suggested a "heartless" streak within evolution. I hoped to find a different explanation.

Several of the physiology graduate students had proposed that the ischemia receptors would do the appropriate thing to save the human's life if blood loss caused the ischemia instead of a blocked artery. If a young caveman suffered a saber tooth tiger attack, these receptors would make his heart race to make up for the blood loss and perhaps save his life. That analysis of the evolutionary benefit of ischemic receptors in the human heart would seem more in line with our concepts of evolution. I liked that explanation.

A few more years passed, and I found myself channel surfing on my television. I hit upon a program presenting the fantastic capabilities of the cheetah, the fastest running animal in the world. The narrator told me that zoologists had learned that the cheetah only runs fast for about half a minute before chest pain makes it stop. The ischemic receptors in the cheetah's heart keep the animal from running until it literally kills itself. Evolution favored ischemic receptors for the cheetah to keep it alive. So perhaps humans have these receptors only because they proved essential for animals from which humans evolved. That may prove the most accurate answer of all.

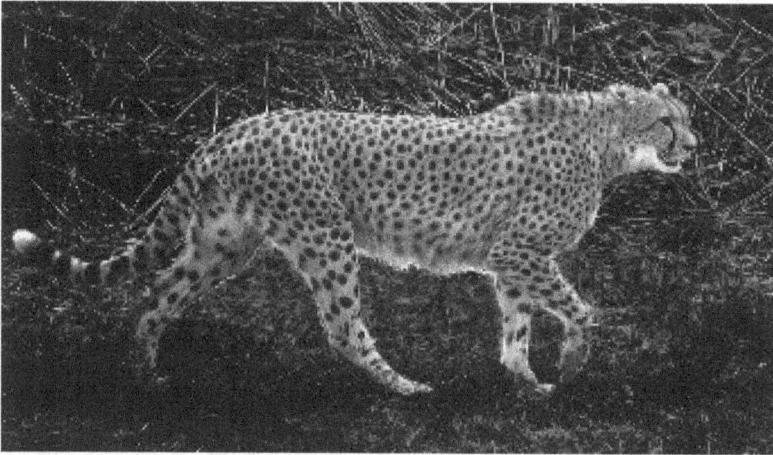

Perspicacity often seems to rely on tracing observations back to how living organisms evolved, just as physicists continuously refer back to the basic rules that govern the way the physical world operates.

If you came up with even a better explanation of why we have these ischemia receptors in our hearts, I would love to hear from you. The human body has some other design flaws that need scrutiny as well.

Chapter 14 What is a fever?

Is it a fever that makes one hot under the collar?
Or is it the shape of the collar that makes one a scholar?
In this chapter we are just going to hoot and holler.

We want more practice at **perspicacity**. We want to better understand how to grow the skill of shrewdness in our study and understanding of medicine. I mentioned that in the study of infectious disease everything seemed to present with fever and malaise. But I cannot recall any teaching on the physiology of fever itself.

Textbooks of pathophysiology explain that fever begins with exposure to pyrogens or endotoxins in the cell walls of invading bacteria or viruses. In response to these endotoxins the human body also releases its own pyrogens, further increasing the fever during its white cell response to these invaders. A long list of potential benefits of fever ensue that appear to help the human in its fight against an infection. Some authorities even argue for caution in the use of medications that reduce a fever. Fever significantly saps the energy of the patient, a consequence especially troublesome in the elderly patient. Still, one can argue that fever benefits the infected individual.

In the television coverage of the COVID-19 Pandemic in 2020, the President of the United States asked an esteemed expert in public health about the role of fever. The expert said that the body mounts a fever to improve its ability to rid itself of the invading infectious agent. And that appears true despite the fact that the fever may reduce the efficiency of some enzymes that have been tuned to work best at a normal body temperature.

In 2005, Scientific American published the words of a physician at Indiana University saying, "The presence of a fever is usually related to stimulation of the body's immune response. Fever...makes the body less favorable as a host for replicating viruses and bacteria, which are temperature sensitive." The article explains that pyrogens trigger the hypothalamus region of the brain to ramp up the body's metabolism to elevate core temperature. They added later in the article without explanation, "Some pyrogens are produced by body tissue; many pathogens also produce pyrogens."

They just slipped that last little phrase into the article, innocently. "Many pathogens also produce pyrogens." Why would pathogens evolve pyrogens on their surface if raising the body's temperature makes the body a less favorable host? Why would pathogens initiate the process of fever? This looks like the sort of riddle we can use to practice **perspicacity**.

When I worked in the medical device industry, I learned for the first time that medical devices that touch patients, especially invasively, must possess the characteristics of sterility, non-pyrogenicity, and non-toxicity. My professors did not emphasize these attributes in their medical school lectures.

I thought that medical devices were either sterile or not, a binary status. Sterile, in my mind, meant free from any bacteria, living organisms, or viable viruses. It shocked me to learn that actually sterile means relatively free of viable organisms. Officially, sterile has a statistical definition.

The FDA tells American manufacturers the statistical level of sterility required for their particular product. The manufacturer puts a known number of bacteria through the sterilization process used for that product and then grows a culture to count the number that survived. A product that comes into contact with breached skin may need a sterility level of 10-6 SAL. SAL stands for "sterility assurance level." The 10-6 number means the probability of a viable microorganism being on the device registers below 1 in 10 raised to the 6th power. Some devices only need a 10-3 SAL.

To claim non-toxic, washings of the device must not significantly injure human cells grown in culture. That means the device cannot have any substance on its surface that disrupts human cell growth in a laboratory.

And finally, non-pyrogenic means that washings of the device injected into a rabbit cannot cause a fever. Pyrogens might come from bacteria that had contaminated the device but were killed during sterilization. The retained material could still cause a fever if left on the device. Thus, pyrogen-free creates a characteristic independent of sterilization.

Getting back to our riddle, we asked why bacteria would evolve the ability to initiate a fever when the fever appears to make their fate less successful. It does make sense that humans, and indeed other animals, evolved a fever response to help them suppress infections. Humans probably inherited that skill in the same manner they inherited ischemia receptors in their heart.

I have not found anyone suggesting an answer to this question in the medical literature. But I would suggest that perhaps the answer lies in the nature of evolution. Evolution cannot improve the performance of an organism engaged in a suicide mission. Evolution only works to enhance a characteristic that makes an organism more likely to replicate itself. Apparently, bacteria do not infect other organisms or humans to enhance the proliferation of their species. Instead, infecting a living organism must be for that particular microbe a terrible mishap. That microbe either kills the host or dies trying, but both outcomes terminate the microbe. The ego of human beings appears to define certain microbes as pathogens, when that definition would certainly never occur to the pathogen. Putting ourselves in the position of the microbe, as Jonas Salk suggested we do, we would not be at all interested in infecting a human. And all this time I thought pathogens were out there just waiting for an opportunity to attack me.

How might one take advantage of this clearer understanding of the motivation of a microbe? I have no idea. Regardless, I think we are improved by taking this journey in thought.

Chapter 15 What are we going to do with genetics?

Emmanuelle Charpentier, Jennifer Dudna, and Feng Zhang,
Have turned CRISPR-Cas9 into a second big bang.
Does this mean we add one more year to med school,
Or will it totally be managed by a computer module?

Courtesy of the basic science community, medical science now has the ability to edit the human genome precisely in a living human being. That ranks as a major game changer. We struggle to have enough imagination to comprehend the eventual impact of this discovery. But we celebrate this triumph that launches a new era in medical care vastly better serving mankind.

Earlier we looked at ultrasonic imaging as a way to allow physicians to find disease and injury in their patients before symptoms present. We could decode a patient's genes for a while, but that ability has not brought huge benefits since we could not correct genetic defects. Now we stand at the beginning of the era of gene therapy. We still need to figure out what we can do safely and ethically, but that will come. We certainly cannot "put the genie of gene editing back in the bottle."

Prior history might suggest that we will create a new medical specialist, perhaps a "Geneticologist." Such a specialist would treat patients with genetic abnormalities and make them normal. That could happen. Alternatively, we might have genetic therapies that physicians in established specialties could incorporate into their work. A third alternative might use the growing capabilities of artificial intelligence to make the capabilities of genetic therapy easily applied. We are going to look more closely at the promise of artificial intelligence in the final chapter. Would you think it ideal for us to harness the power of new technologies in our future to make all health practitioners alike, as was the case in the Wild West? Perhaps then medical practitioners could treat all human ailments and do so with equal ability. Should that be our goal? That seems the ideal way to make health care universally available.

Some might want to draw a line to say that no one should fix certain irregularities in our genes. That may prove a difficult issue to resolve. If born with the genes predicting an adult height of five feet tall, should taller become an option? Should the height needed for a career in professional basketball become a choice or remain a chance event?

CRISPR-Cas9 gives the medical science community the capability to create an agent dubbed "a gene drive." A gene drive puts instructions into the organism's genes to edit the genes of future generations, so a genetic edit recurs in all progeny. Armed with this ability all sorts of amazing disease prevention strategies become possible. For example, CRISPR-Cas9 could be used to eliminate Lyme Disease by modifying the genetics of the nine small animals known to serve as a reservoir. We could make them no longer a reservoir for the Borrelia spiral bacteria that causes Lyme disease. Do we prefer to take this step? A vaccination exists for dogs and humans. The initial human vaccine seems to have side effects which discourage its use. Permethrin can be used on outdoor clothing to ward off ticks. And early treatment with an antibiotic can usually stop a bite from progressing to the disease. So far, the alternatives seem less risky than using a genetic fix that might have unexpected irreversible consequences that would prove difficult to rule out.

Obviously, it makes sense to use powerful new tools cautiously. Having said that, no one can expect launching a career in medical science today without expecting that CRISPR-Cas9 will drastically change how we manage disease and injuries.

Did you notice the word "injuries" crept into that last sentence? How could CRISPR-Cas9 do anything about an injury? It appears that geneticists are getting very close to understanding how a lizard might have the ability to regrow its tail after a traumatic amputation, but humans cannot do the same even for trauma to our little toe. You might wake up one morning to find that CRISPR-Cas9 has changed that situation. And perhaps that means we might grow a new kidney or liver as well.

I certainly wanted to play professional basketball at one point in my youth. I had becoming an FBI agent as a backup plan. Somehow, I never got close to either career. Now, as a retired older American, my primary care physician constantly suggests that I should probably get more exercise. But I tend toward laziness. This situation might suggest a tiny exercise in **perspicacity**, that might neighbor on genetics indirectly.

If you avoid my laziness and do get some strenuous exercise your body apparently increases a chemical in the plasma called anandamide. This agent apparently creates some degree of euphoria that gets some people hooked on running marathons and such. But on a more fundamental level we all know that if we lift weights today our muscles grow bigger and stronger over an ensuing period of time. Muscle cells must have some way to remember that you made them work hard yesterday. But how does that work? I figured that the muscle fiber must manufacture a protein in response to exercise that stayed around to encourage muscles to get bigger and stronger.

In 1997, Professor Jin Lee at Johns Hopkins discovered that in mice this process seems to work in the opposite direction. A regulatory molecule may inhibit the genes that grow muscles. Lee's research led to a protein-based therapy for growing muscle that I had in my own imagination previously named the "Exercise Molecule for the Lazy." Apparently, work continues on such a drug in earnest to help treat muscular dystrophies. Initial trials of Lee's myostatin inhibitor had dangerous side effects in some healthy volunteers. I feel like **perspicacity** led me to predict this drug would come to my rescue long before I heard of Professor Lee's work. I still have hope as I lounge on my sofa.

Chapter 16 What Should We Expect from Artificial Intelligence?

Every American warship boasts an autonomous gun,
That will shoot down a missile the ship sure can't outrun.
Artificial intelligence keeps making more of our decisions,
And soon we hope it can prevent all those car collisions.

Perspicacity insists that we view the growth of artificial intelligence as a means to prevent mistakes in health care. It should also accelerate medical research. Indeed, it promises to make the world more capable with a spectrum of skills we cannot begin to list. In short, we hope that generalized artificial intelligence can bring great opportunities to mankind. Many have voiced fear that computers growing "smarter" than humans will bring the death of mankind, literally. That legitimate concern will not stop progress, so instead, we need to remain perspicacious. We need to choose our world's leadership carefully. We must shrewdly insist that we nourish honor and caring in all of human society. At the same time, we must oppress avarice aggressively. Would it not prove ironic if generalized artificial intelligence afforded us the most effective means to carry out those noble objectives?

I used the phrase generalized artificial intelligence. Artificial intelligence has grown an array of divisions. Some systems developed to mimic human smartness in specific tasks we call "narrow or focused AI." Machines that learn and attempt to mimic humans more broadly we refer to as "strong AI" or "generalized AI." I have imagined that physicians and other medical care providers in the future would have a device similar to a hearing aid. This device would listen to oral speech and conversations and, when appropriate, whisper suggestions into the care provider's ear. You can easily imagine such a device could search all the world's knowledge for information. It could organize treatment protocols, such as those Brent James developed, and whisper valuable cues moment-to-moment into the practitioner's ear. I imagine that it might listen in to provider to patient conversations and be prepared to suggest an alternative test, diagnosis, question, or treatment. I see the provider in the future saying something like, "Let me think for a moment about the situation you have described." That statement would prompt the whispering AI to make a suggestion. After all, AI never forgets, thinks a thousand times faster than a human, does not need sleep, never takes a vacation, and seems reasonably resistant to malice unless commanded to go in that direction. What a wonderful, loyal assistant to have!

When we compare the speed with which a human and a computer can multiply two large numbers together, we get a ratio in the thousands, if not higher. Computers have grown faster and faster. Years ago, I read that if we could work as fast as a computer, our normal speed of typing to the machine would seem as though we were hitting one key about every month or two.

The computing machine I am using to write at this moment has a clock speed of 3.5 billion cycles per second. I believe I am operating much slower. The nerves in my body have a maximum transmission velocity of less than 268 miles per hour compared to the speed of light for electrical signals in a wire at 186,282 miles per second. The makes the signals moving about in my computer travel 2,502,296 times faster.

Comparing a computer to human performance in general gets tricky. But a computer that can research a topic with the skill of a human would seem to offer a great advance. A computer assistant working in real time conversing in English could enhance patient care immensely, and that capability appears to loom on the horizon.

The growth of artificial intelligence would potentially drive many human careers into extinction during the coming century. Medical specialist in radiology have expressed concern for their future even now. Artificial intelligence based on "deep learning" algorithms has demonstrated before the year 2020 the ability to read diagnostic imaging more reliably accurate than can human radiologists. One can imagine that machines will in the future outperform numerous medical care specialties. Humans appear to outperform machines in trust and bonding. Those skills have great importance in the healing arts. But one would have difficulty arguing that the information management talents of digital machines will not eventually improve medical care in virtually all of its dimensions.

Quite likely the capabilities of artificial intelligence will allow medical practitioners to minister to patients more reliably with fewer years of training. I would hope that humans will be free to put more time and energy into their unique caring talents and enjoy longer and more satisfying careers. Artificial intelligence holds the potential of vastly reducing the need for human labor to support the necessities of a comfortable life for all people as it expands the productivity of a society. So, people could have more time for the pursuit of kindness and creativity. What could prove better?

In conversations with friends on the subject of artificial intelligence, I find people have worries that human programmers will introduce dangerous bias into the systems they build. Also, uncertainty abounds over the safety of building systems that can think like humans but thousands of times faster. Every step science takes to advances our capabilities comes with risk of unintended consequences and dangers. Worry over the dangers should remain. People must have an understanding of what these systems do and stay involved in society's decisions.

A species of artificial intelligence called "deep learning" has created spectacular achievements going into 2020 that either excite or frighten. The response seems to depend upon one's confidence in the future. This particular type of AI attempts to copy the way our own brain functions. Humans have billions of neurons. Each neuron constantly adds up the impulses arriving on its surface and decides, based on that sum, whether to fire off an impulse itself or not do so. If the arriving stimuli reaches a threshold level in a specific neuron, it fires and sends an impulse to many hundreds of other neurons. Each time it fires, the neuron adjusts its sensitivity to each one of the hundreds of neurons that caused it to fire. Researchers have dubbed the scheme used for these adjustments "back propagation."

You might best understand "back propagation" by imagining a child learning to recognize the letters of the alphabet. A parent or teacher presents a letter. The child makes an identification and the instructor either corrects an error or rewards a correct identification. In some manner the instructor's response has to translate into an adjustment of the sensitivity of all the inputs to each neuron involved in the recognition so that the frequency of correct letter identifications keeps climbing. We call that process education. The child keeps adjusting the sensitivity to each input of every neuron constantly because we keep learning and keep remembering throughout our lives.

Programmers of artificial intelligence essentially keep working at the efficiency and stability of "back propagation." I find it hard to imagine how social bias would enter into that process. On the other hand, bias seems to enter into the process of teaching from the choice of examples of content we wish the intelligent system to learn. You would probably agree that we all learn bias not from the mechanics of how our neurons adjust themselves (the programmer's role), but from the information presented to us to learn (the instructor's role).

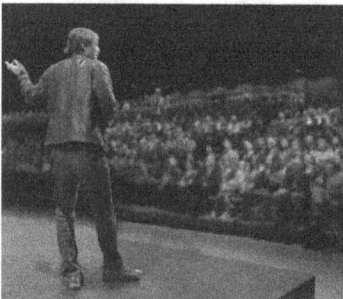

Artificial intelligence guru, Dr. Max Tegmark at MIT, has suggested that humans will perhaps drive improvements to "back propagation" for about another decade. Then artificial intelligence systems may do a better job of inventing the subsequent iterations. In that way, artificial intelligence should improve itself exponentially into the years ahead.

As we think about such a future, we ask ourselves, "Will such systems develop self-awareness?" I arrive at my answer to that question in a backward fashion. I cannot see any reason why they would not. Some aspects of self-awareness in humans seems to come from our sense of touch and our ability to feel pain. Giving those capabilities to generalized artificial intelligence systems would constitute a choice a human designer would need to make.

I have noticed that many of my friends have trouble separating artificial intelligence from robotics. Robots have quite different attributes. Both can exist separately, although I can imagine the two advances coming together at some point to inhabit this world. If we make the robots into super strong, fast machines, then we have created a new set of issues and concerns that we may wish to postpone. Cyborgs intimidate me.

The future just keeps coming. I have gotten to an age that makes me eager to see what comes next, but not too concerned that I have to live through all of the consequences. I can certainly appreciate younger people, especially my grandchildren, need to have a different perspective and level of concern.

We are talking about the medical sciences, and the coming of generalized artificial intelligence appears to offer great dividends both for the delivery of care and the development of better care. I feel that people will continue to prefer to have humans care for them. But we should not care that machines double check to prevent errors, and when appropriate, suggest therapeutic options humans may not have considered. We probably will not object to leading longer, healthier lives. I am optimistic.

Chapter 17 The Culmination

Sgt. Joe Friday says, "Just the facts, Ma'am."
That's all you may need to pass the exam.
But to make our world a better place,
Please practice perspicacity for the human race.

In the beginning we talked about a novel way of teaching a course that starts with a review of the entire topic and ends with an integration of the important concepts.

The time has arrived for the integration. We have made the case that the fire hose of information in medical education can easily put out the fire of curiosity. We want to avoid that outcome. Possibly, people with a passion for deductive sciences have some degree of immunity. Those people naturally dwell on the foundational principles that make sense of what they see.

We all are born with curiosity. We start asking why as soon as we learn that word. Humans keep asking why until something beats that habit out of us. Perhaps this book has heightened your awareness of your natural inclination. If you plan to study a topic in the medical sciences, I hope to have rekindled your natural instinct to ask why.

Facts do not become knowledge until we understand why the world behaves as it does. Persistently asking "how come" will save lives.

You have been reading examples of insights. Some chapters have suggested tips for seeking the reasons behind what the professors teach. My father taught economics at the college level. He sincerely wanted his students to fashion unique viewpoints on issues. Still, he complained that his sophomores wanted to debate before they had learned the meaning of the words they wanted to spout. Nonetheless, he loved the process of nurturing their sophistication of thought and analysis.

I believe he would wholeheartedly approve of this book's objective. I am pushing, as he would have, for future healthcare professionals to search incessantly for the reasons behind concepts and procedures. Trainees must still learn the vocabulary of words and concepts required to interpret and communicate, and then ask why.

In my third year of medical school, everyone did a clinical rotation in internal medicine, featuring an oral examination in the final week. A clinical faculty member who had not worked with our specific team conducted the exam. Each student provided a list of patients he or she had treated during the rotation to guide the choice of topics for the examination. My examination started with a discussion of a patient with new-onset Type II Diabetes admitted with dangerously elevated blood sugar. I was eager to talk about everything we did for him, how it went, and why we elected each treatment. Instead, the examiner asked me how many Americans have diabetes? I knew the disease affected millions of people, especially in an obese population. But I did not know the number. I said I did not know the number.

The examiner chastised me. "If you have read about and studied the condition you treated, you must have run across the prevalence of diabetes in our nation. Why don't you know how many people have this condition?" I could not give him a number, and he would not move on. He insisted this knowledge was essential because common problems show up commonly and demand expert attention. I took my beating and never got an opportunity to talk about what we had done for the patient. The examiner then went on to another case, and again I was grilled on details that seemed more aligned with demographics than pathophysiology.

I remember that experience as a total misreading of what the teacher deemed vital in the lesson content. I had never experienced such a misconception in my basic science and engineering courses. I often had not learned my lessons thoroughly, but I never felt I had studied the wrong material.

One of my classmates told me that he had flipped back to the first page several times during a particularly tough written medical school examination to make sure he had not gotten a test intended for a different course. I laughed, but I also knew what he meant exactly.

We have been encouraging students pursuing careers in healthcare to practice **perspicacity,** mindful of the tradition of medical education to stress memorization of billowing details. The emphasis in this book on the visualization of the foundational mechanisms behind the details cannot excuse the need to learn those details. Instead, we are saying the student must learn the details, but not forget to look behind the curtain. We offer hope that technology will soon find a way to provide the reliable, germane details to us at high speed. Then **perspicacity** can spring freely into action to orchestrate our treatments into the most compassionate symphony of care one human being can offer another.

The novel way of teaching we discussed in Chapter 1 requires that I go one more step. I have the obligation of pulling together themes that we have discussed to suggest how they foster a better path for humanity. Is this possible? Of course. Otherwise, you would deserve a refund on the purchase price of this slender book.

We devoted several pages to the pivotal role of the enzyme in the creation of life on this planet called Earth. Evolution teaches that enzymes arrived by chance, not by intent. Similarly, the complexity of all life we believe came about from the natural selection of random events and not by deliberate choices. We discussed the importance of control systems at work in the physiology of life. We again concluded that they emerged by natural selection. Therefore, extinction constituted a critical process in the advancement of biological capabilities for both plants and animals.

But what about the future? Are we moving ever closer to an inflection point in evolution? By an inflection point, I mean a change in the trajectory of the future of living organisms. Think for a moment what it would take to replace evolution with biological enhancement by intention.

Now that you have become fully **perspicacious**, suppose we put you entirely in charge of the future of all life forms. What capabilities do you need to replace the brutality of evolution? I trust you agree that evolution has proven itself brutal to the core.

Please stop and ponder that question for a moment before you contaminate your ideas with mine.

I would want two new capabilities before I forge a radical new path into the future. I want the ability to design new enzymes and the ability to teach living organisms how to manufacture those enzymes.

The second ability has mostly arrived, as discussed in Chapter 15. Nessa Carey explains the state of gene editing thoroughly in her book entitled *Hacking the Code of Life.* However, designing enzymes appears still unsolved.

Daniel Bolon and Stephen Mayo wrote two decades ago on forging steps toward the computational design of protein enzymes for industrial and medical applications. Nature has solved this problem by trial-and-error selection of randomly generated candidates. Instead, we want the ability to computationally describe the task we want the enzyme to carry out. Then we want a computer to figure out the structure of the protein necessary to catalyze that reaction. The designed protein should fold itself precisely into the scaffold shape required to support the desired chemical reaction. This computational approach seems an objective clearly in need of artificial intelligence. We know how to convert the protein sequence into the genetic code that a cell would require to assemble the enzyme.

Scientists are knocking at the door of enzyme design. When that door opens, life on Earth changes its trajectory.

You may have read about the magical properties of graphene. Graphene makes possible supercapacitors to replace slowly charging batteries and space elevators to lift us gently into orbit in space. Figuring out how to make graphene in large quantities represents yet another door to a very different world separate from biology. The list of potential uses for graphene seems endless. The challenge of graphene lies in getting carbon atoms to link together in a one-atom-thick membrane. They want very much to belong to that structure, but they resist aligning themselves thus. And we need them to align that way in vast quantities. That sure sounds like an enzyme problem to me.

Have I done it? Have I given you a culmination that pulls together aspects of our discussion of **perspicacity**? Have I proven the importance of asking why again and again? Have I encouraged you to think harder? If I have come close, I am proud. Dr. Hill pushed me unmercifully to get us to this point. I thank him for that.

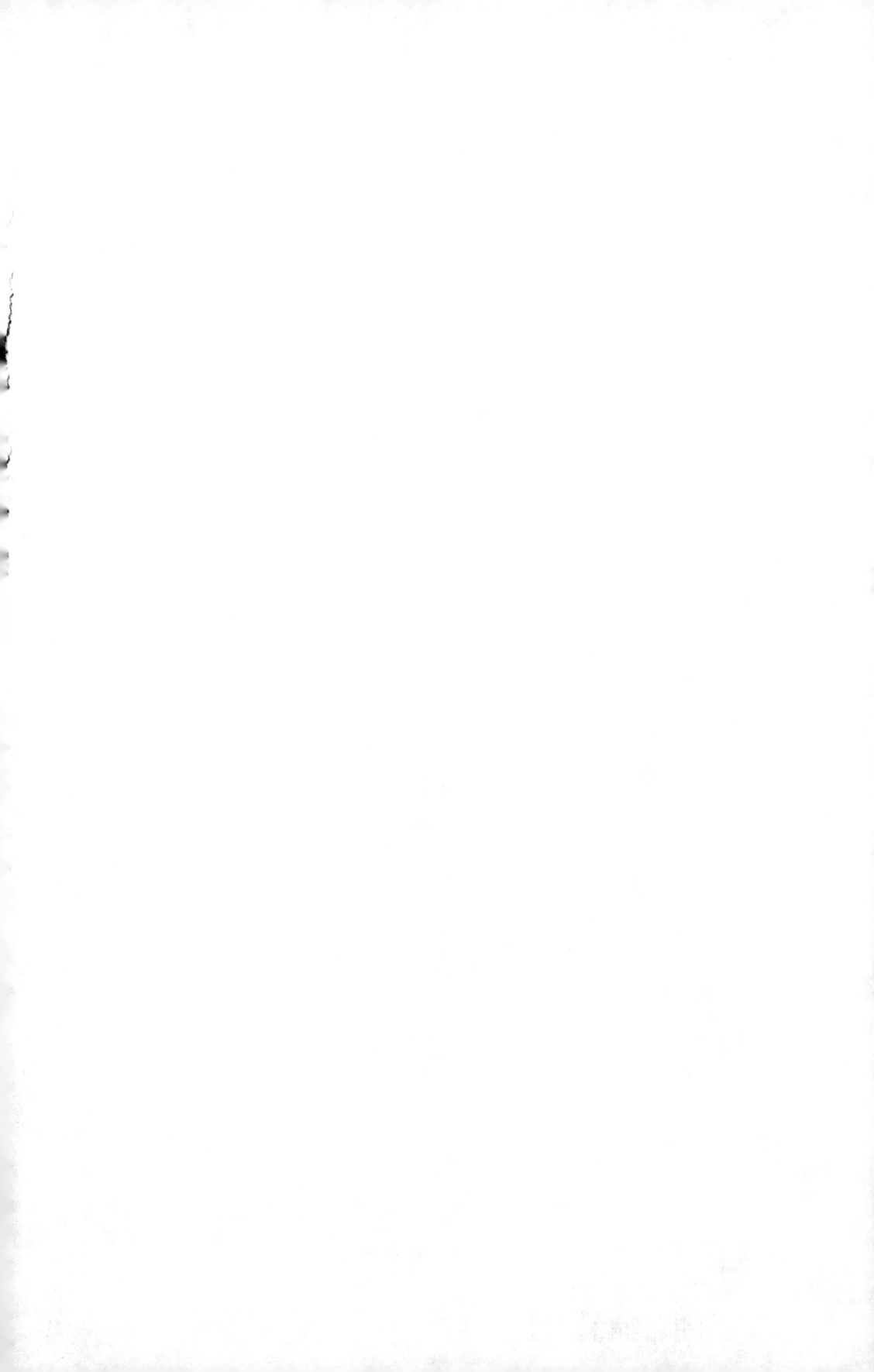

www.ingramcontent.com/pod-product-compliance
Lightning Source LLC
Chambersburg PA
CBHW050230270326
41914CB00003BA/641